THE POC

PeriMenopause

by Sahar Hooti

The first interactive women's health book - blending ancient wisdom, modern science, and self-care

Best wishes,

Sahar x

The Pocket Guide to PeriMenopause

First edition

Published by Hooti Press, Portsmouth, United Kingdom

www.acucareclinic.co.uk

Published by Hooti Press, Portsmouth, United Kingdom

www.acucareclinic.co.uk

A CIP catalogue record for this book is available from the British Library.

ISBN (Paperback): 978-1-9192670-0-5

ISBN (eBook): 978-1-9192670-1-2

Cover design by Roxana Hooti

Illustrations by Roxana Hooti

Edited by Leanne Curran

TRADEMARK & COPYRIGHT NOTICE

"I started working with Sahar during a time when I felt like I was losing myself. Her approach - both in clinic and online - helped me understand what was happening in my body and how to support it. The tools she gave me became part of my everyday life. This book is like having her in your corner, cheering you on. You're in good hands."

~ Emily, 46.

"Sahar's approach to women's health, combining ancient and modern medicine, has genuinely transformed my health and sense of self. She has helped me understand the root causes of issues and given me practical tools to help manage them. This book epitomises her approach - kind, holistic and effective."

~ Leanne, 38.

For all the women of history and the women of today who endured this transition in silence. What was once taboo no longer is. For my mum, who came through her own transition with courage and grace. For my dad, whose quiet creativity inspired me to write. And for my patients, who remind me daily that this journey is never walked alone.

DEAR READER

I didn't expect to be writing this book while walking through PeriMenopause myself. But life has a way of turning your profession into your purpose.

This book was born from both experience and heartbreak. Over 20 years ago, someone I love deeply spiralled during PeriMenopause. Lost in symptoms no one talked about, let alone understood. The fear, the rage, the hopelessness was terrifying to witness. Yet she was far from alone.

In the UK alone, around 13 million women are navigating PeriMenopause or menopause right now. That's roughly one-third of the female population. Globally, by the end of 2025, over 1 billion women are expected to be in menopause, and millions more in the years leading up to it. Yet so many are still left in the dark, enduring symptoms for an average of 4-8 years*. So I wrote this to say: we don't have to suffer in silence anymore.

This is for every woman who ever questioned her sanity in the middle of the night. For the ones who kept smiling while slowly falling apart. For the women who were told to get on with it (and did) but paid the price in silence.

This is for you.

The Pocket Guide to PeriMenopause is unlike anything I could find when I needed it most, and it's the first interactive women's health book dedicated to PeriMenopause. It's a practical, science-informed self-care companion built from my clinical experience, cultural heritage, and personal journey.

Everything in these pages comes from decades of hands-on work with women and draws on thousands of years of Traditional Chinese Medicine. It hasn't been through lab trials. It doesn't need to. When something consistently supports real women in real life, that's evidence worth trusting.

Inside you'll find Advanced Acupressure, including my Press-Pulsate-Pause Method™ (also known as the PPP Method™), healing breath rituals, aromatherapy, and affirmations, woven together with the quiet, stubborn wisdom passed down by the Persian women who raised me.

Think of it as your witty best friend and trusted Acupuncture Practitioner in one. A book you can throw in your bag, or slip into a large dress pocket (and if you find one with a massive pocket, tag me, because who doesn't love that?). Reach for it when you feel overwhelmed, lost, or just need someone to say: You don't need fixing. You need understanding.

This isn't a "how to survive" manual. This is a rebel book of real self-care in a chaotic hormonal world.

It's a privilege to be alive in an age where we finally get to talk about this. And it's an honour to walk this part of the path with you.

With love, and a reminder that you've always had the power,

Sahar x

PREFACE

The Book That Helped Me Back to Myself.

I began writing this book in September 2024 with a clear purpose: to empower women with practical, science-backed self-care tools for navigating PeriMenopause. What I didn't realise then was just how personal that mission was about to become.

In May 2025, just weeks before my 44th birthday, I received my official diagnosis: I was in PeriMenopause. The symptoms had been showing up quietly, then loudly, for years. Looking back, I now see they started as early as age 36 but, like so many women, I didn't have the language, the diagnosis, or the space to fully understand what was happening. Until now.

So while I began writing this book as a practitioner, I finished it as a patient too.

Brain fog, anxiety, forgetfulness, hot flushes, night sweats and still, I wrote. There were moments I forgot what I was writing mid-sentence, and days I wanted to pack it all away and do something easier. But this book anchored me. It helped me remember who I am. It helped me heal.

Writing it reminded me of everything I already teach. It helped me practise what I preach.

The Press-Pulsate-Pause Method™, the breathwork, the affirmations, the aromatherapy rituals, I didn't just write them for you. I used them myself. And they worked.

So no, this isn't a book I wish someone else had written. This is the book I needed and I wrote it while walking through the very thing I was writing about.

I've worked with women for over 20 years, and this book honours every patient who's ever sat in front of me, unsure of what's happening to her body. It honours the women who came before us: the ones who suffered in silence, who were dismissed or misdiagnosed, who lost parts of themselves because no one gave them the words, the care, or the space to understand what was happening.

One of those women was someone I love deeply. Her struggle was heartbreaking to witness, and back then, there was no book, no language, no support. Only confusion and despair.

This book exists to help make sure that never happens again.

Writing it has reminded me that healing doesn't require perfection. Just presence.

So take your time. Breathe. Flip to the chapter you need most and let this book be your toolkit, your comfort, and your call to reclaim yourself - one page at a time.

Why Persian Wisdom Lives in These Pages

I was born in Iran during the Iran-Iraq war, raised between Iran, Australia, and England, and shaped by the stories of the women who came before me - my mother, my grandmother, my aunts.

Whether we were gathered over tea, sharing food, or deep in quiet conversation, there was always a Persian saying offered to soothe, guide, or ground the moment. For every emotion, every struggle, every joy, there was a line of poetry or philosophy that somehow made sense of it all.

These sayings aren't just words. They carry comfort, clarity, and perspective - much like acupuncture and Traditional Chinese Medicine. For me, Persian wisdom is a form of meditation. A way to return to stillness. A way to remember who we are.

Like a balm for the soul, they offer meaning when life feels chaotic.

That's why throughout this book, you'll find these sayings carefully placed like heirlooms passed down through generations. You don't need to be Persian to feel their power. Their essence is universal.

Note

This book is built on decades of clinical practice, Traditional Chinese Medicine, and real-world experience with women in PeriMenopause. It's a self-care companion, not a replacement for a one-to-one consultation or medical advice. Always work alongside a qualified health professional when needed and trust your own body as your greatest guide.

INTRODUCTION

You're Not Sick - You're Taking Control

Welcome, PM Warrior.

Yes, you! The Prime Minister of your body and hormones. Congratulations on taking the first step towards mastering PeriMenopause like a boss.

Let's get something straight from the start: you're not "sick," "broken," or losing your mind. You're in a transition and one that's often misunderstood, dismissed, or, worse, completely ignored. This is your time to take the reins. This journey isn't about just surviving PeriMenopause. It's about thriving through it.

In these pages, you're going to become the CEO of your health. You're the boss here, not your hormones.

Why I spell it "PeriMenopause" - You'll notice I capitalise it throughout this book because it's not just a phase. It's a power shift. A full-body rebellion. And the "PM" in PM Warrior? That's you, stepping into your next level.

Here's the Truth

PeriMenopause isn't an illness. It's a hormonal shift, and with the right support, it's entirely manageable. I'm not promising miracles. This book won't pretend to "fix" you (because you're not broken), but it will help you:

- Make sense of what's happening in your body.
- Reclaim control over your symptoms.
- Feel like yourself again. Clear, confident, and calm.

We'll do it together, using advanced acupressure, aromatherapy, breath rituals, affirmations, and holistic tools drawn from both ancient wisdom and modern research.

What You'll Find Inside

No, we won't cover every PeriMenopausal symptom but we will focus on the ones I see most often in clinic such as:

- Mood swings.
- Sleep disturbances.
- Brain fog.
- Skin and digestive changes.
- Hormonal crashes that seem to come out of nowhere.

For each, I'll walk you through what's happening and what you can do about it.

You'll also see references to the Hooti Method™, a clinical, experience-based framework I've developed over years of work with women's hormonal health. It brings together traditional wisdom, targeted acupressure, and holistic science to offer results you can feel.

You'll learn how to use the Press-Pulsate-Pause Method™ (PPP Method™), essential oil rituals, lifestyle tweaks, and small daily shifts that make a big difference.

By the end, you'll feel clearer, more in control, and supported every step of the way.

How to Use This Book and What it's All About

This guide is designed to be actionable, not overwhelming. Each chapter is structured to help you:

- Look up your concerns in the table of contents.
- Try practical techniques for immediate relief.

- Use QR codes to follow video demos (no guessing!).
- Track your progress to learn what works for you.

And if you're not sure where to begin with the videos and extra resources, head to the appendix. There you'll find a complete section with everything you need in one place.

A Word on AcuWarrior™

Before the pandemic, I envisioned AcuWarrior™ as a way to honour the ancient practitioners of acupuncture. Those who passed down these healing traditions, even when they were silenced.

Now, AcuWarrior™ is a registered trademark, and you'll see "AcuWarrior™ Tips" throughout this book. These aren't just wellness hacks. They're part of a living lineage. A bridge between old and new. And you, reader, are part of that bridge.

Affirmations: More Than Fluff

I used to roll my eyes at affirmations until the pandemic hit. Lockdown had me scribbling hopeful words on sticky notes and posting them around the house. Before long, I was handing out personalised affirmations to my patients alongside aromatherapy blends. And the feedback? Beautiful. Transformational.

Here's the science: affirmations help rewire the brain. They strengthen new thought pathways, reduce stress, and support emotional resilience. Each chapter in this book opens or closes with one. Keep them. Speak them. Let them remind you: you're not alone, and you're not powerless.

The Science of Gratitude

Gratitude isn't just a feel-good trend. It boosts dopamine, lowers cortisol, and literally rewires the brain. Towards the end of each chapter, I'll invite you to jot down one or two things you've noticed, small moments you can be thankful for. Tiny wins matter.

Gratitude shifts your hormones, supports your nervous system, and helps you ride the waves with more ease.

A Quick Word About Sharing This Book

Although this guide is written for you, it's also meant to be shared. You'll find pages and charts throughout that aren't just helpful for you. They're designed to be shown to the people around you. Your partner. Your family. Your friends. Anyone in your circle who cares about you. Even your kids (if age-appropriate).

Why? Because PeriMenopause isn't something you should have to explain alone, or, worse, suffer through in silence while everyone else is wondering what's going on. If PeriMenopause is going to be normalised, it needs to be understood. Not just by women going through it, but by everyone who walks beside us.

Let's Get Started

By the time you close this book, I hope you'll feel:

- Stronger in your body.
- Calmer in your mind.
- More connected to yourself.

You haven't lost yourself. You're coming back to her. Your body isn't your enemy. It's your ride-or-die.

And PeriMenopause? She's not here to ruin you. She's here to wake you up.

Rituals, Routines & Hormone Rewiring

This book is small enough to fit in your bag, but bold enough to change how you show up for yourself. You don't need a full hour, a fancy yoga mat, or a degree in Chinese medicine. You just need a few minutes a day and a willingness to try. This is about making self-care realistic, not romanticised.

Each chapter gives you tools you can actually use with no pressure to follow a fixed order. You get to choose the rhythm. This is your space.

The Press-Pulsate-Pause Method™

The Press-Pulsate-Pause Method™ (Also known as the PPP Method™) is my signature Advanced Acupressure ritual.It's short, potent, and supported by quick QR demos.You'll learn how to use these points to rebalance hormones, ease stress, and come home to your body in just two minutes a day.

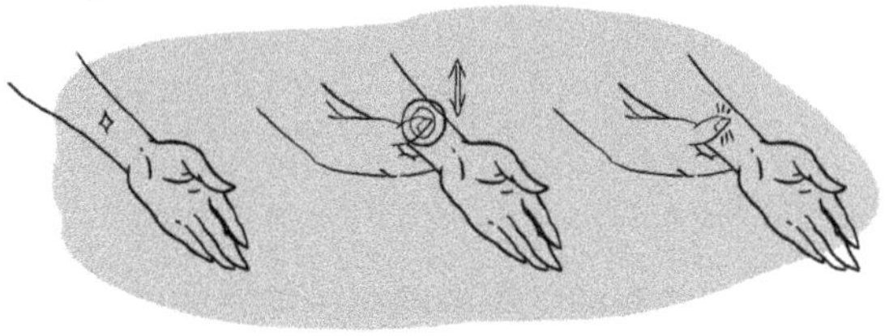

AcuWarrior™ Tip: It doesn't matter which side of your body you start treatment with but I start from the right side because I always like to think we are always right (joking obviously, but that's what I like to do).

Aromatherapy & Breathwork

Each chapter includes an optional essential oil suggestion and breath ritual, designed to support sleep, mood, energy, or emotional reset. You'll learn to pair breath with scent to create mini rituals that fit your life.

"Breathe in through your nose. Exhale through your mouth. Trust that your body wants to support you."

Affirmations That Actually Land

Not fluffy. Not forced. These are neuroscience-backed mantras for rewiring thought patterns and they're woven in naturally, often near the end of chapters or after a key practice.

Persian Wisdom:

"Words carry seeds. Plant them wisely."

Symptom Tracking

You'll be shown how to use the Hooti Method™ Symptom Tracker to notice patterns without obsessing.

You're not unpredictable. You're cyclical and awareness helps you reclaim that rhythm.

Gratitude Prompts (That Aren't Cringey)

Gratitude can shift your chemistry, literally. Each chapter ends with a gentle, no-pressure prompt to help you reflect, reframe, and lift your emotional baseline. You might even do this while cupping your hands around a favourite mug. For me, a moment of Sahar's Chai™ is often where reflection begins.

AcuWarrior™ Tips

Think of these as laser-focused nudges drawn from Traditional Medicine and my 20+ years in the clinic. They're here to help you strengthen your self-care and lead with clarity, not just cope.

QR Codes & Demo Links

No guesswork. No overwhelm. Just short, simple video walkthroughs to show you each ritual in your own time.

Repeat. Reset. Reclaim.

This book isn't about doing it all. It's about doing what works with consistency and compassion.

When life feels loud, come back to this. This isn't failure. It's a transition.

Healing Breath Ritual

Ritual steps:

- Close your eyes.
- Breathe in through your nose for 4.
- Hold for 4.
- Exhale gently through your mouth for 6.
- Repeat the affirmation below.

Affirmation

"I am not here to fix myself. I am here to meet myself more deeply."

This is the season of becoming. My power has always been within me.

Repeat the affirmation above, trusting that your cells are ready to support you and not sabotage you.

Persian Wisdom

"Preserve the soul gently, like something handed down."

جان را به یادگاری نگه دار

Transliteration: Jān rā be yādgāri negah dār

Meaning: A gentle reminder to care for your inner self - not as something to fix, but as something to honour. Your soul is not a problem to solve. It's a legacy to tend to.

Let's begin.

CHAPTER 1
"Am I PeriMenopausal?"

So, how do you actually know if you're in PeriMenopause? You've probably Googled it at 2 a.m., wondering if it's "normal" to wake up feeling like a furnace or to cry because a dog ad on telly made your heart melt. Well, you're in the right place.

PeriMenopause is the lead-up to menopause. A transitional phase where your hormones shift and symptoms show up, sometimes quietly, sometimes loudly. It's often misunderstood, misdiagnosed, or dismissed. But here's the truth:

You're not going mad. You're just changing.

Let's Bust a Common Myth

Menopause is not a phase, it's a milestone. It marks exactly one day: the 12-month anniversary of your last period. Everything before that is PeriMenopause. Everything after is PostMenopause. But somewhere along the way, the word menopause became a shortcut for everything hormonal. No wonder it's confusing. No wonder support gets lost in translation.

Let's clear this up so we can finally talk about what's really happening, and get the help we actually need. It's not a phase. It's not your whole identity. It's a moment that deserves the right words and better conversations.

You're not overreacting. You're re-educating and that's powerful. Now let's get you the tools to back it up.

Signs You Might Be in PeriMenopause

Real talk. Here's what to watch for, straight from women who've been there.

No clinical jargon. Just the truth.

1. Your Periods Have Gone Off Script

Maybe your periods are playing hide-and-seek. Or maybe they've arrived with more drama than a season finale cliffhanger.

Whether they've gone AWOL or become erratic, this is usually the first sign your hormones are doing something new.

2. Hot Flushes & Night Sweats

You're sweating like you've just run a marathon but you haven't moved an inch. Hot flushes often strike out of nowhere, and night sweats can turn your bed into a swimming pool.

Glamorous? Not quite. Common? Absolutely.

3. Mood Swings & Rage

You go from peaceful to possessed in 30 seconds flat. That sharp rage? It's not "just stress", it's your hormones talking. Think of it as your body waving a big red flag saying: "Please pay attention."

PeriRage is real. It's linked to declining oestrogen and its effect on serotonin (your feel-good hormone). It doesn't mean you're broken. It means your chemistry is shifting.

Other Common Signs

- Trouble sleeping (hello, 3 a.m. thoughts).
- Brain fog or memory blips ("Umm… what's your name again?").
- Low libido or vaginal dryness.
- Weight gain around the waist ("yes, I hear you sigh").
- Increased headaches or migraines.

How Can You Be Sure?

Here's the tricky part: there's no single test that says "yes, you're in PeriMenopause." It's a diagnosis based on patterns and how you feel.

1. Talk to Your GP

In the UK, blood tests aren't always the first route. In the UK, GPs, nurses or pharmacists can advise on PeriMenopause and refer you onwards. They usually assess based on age, history & symptoms, not just hormones. Still, a good GP will help you rule out other causes.

2. Blood Tests (Sometimes)

If tests are offered, they may check:

- FSH (follicle-stimulating hormone)
- Oestrogen levels

But remember: these fluctuate daily, so a normal reading doesn't rule anything out.

3. Rule Out Other Conditions

Thyroid issues, fibroids, anaemia, or B12 deficiency can mimic PeriMenopause symptoms. Make sure you're not missing something else.

4. NHS Menopause Clinics

You're not on your own. The NHS now offers specialist menopause services in some regions. Here's what you need to know:

- Some clinics were launched as early as 2022, e.g. Somerset and Liverpool hubs.
- Referral routes: Typically through your GP, who can refer you if:

  - Your symptoms are complex.

  - HRT management is unclear.

  - Specialist advice is needed on alternatives.

- In some areas, group digital consultations are available.
- These services may require specialist GP training and can be on a referral or triage basis. Waiting times vary.

Ask your GP directly about a referral to your local NHS Menopause Clinic or "Menopause Hub". Some regions allow virtual consultations, and services are steadily expanding to fill gaps.

Quick Checklist: Are You in PeriMenopause?

▢ Tick any that apply:

▢ My periods are irregular or changing

▢ I've had hot flushes or night sweats

▢ I've noticed intense mood swings or sudden rage

▢ I struggle with sleep

▢ I feel foggy or forgetful

▢ I've experienced vaginal dryness or a drop in libido

▢ I've gained weight around the waist

▢ I get more headaches or migraines than usual

If you ticked three or more, then welcome! This might be PeriMenopause. You're not alone. And you're not powerless.

What You Can Do Next

1. Start Tracking Your Symptoms

Awareness = empowerment. Start tracking your symptoms daily or weekly. Patterns will emerge.

You'll learn how to use the Hooti Method™ Symptom Tracker later in the book so no need to do it perfectly now.

2. Book That Appointment

If this chapter felt a little too familiar then it's time to talk to your GP. If they suggest bloods or seem unsure, you can ask to be referred to a Menopause Clinic.

And if you're dismissed? Advocate louder. You know your body better than anyone.

3. Consider Your Options

This book focuses on natural support including the Press-Pulsate-Pause Method™, aromatherapy, acupressure, breath rituals, and more.

But there are medical options too, like HRT. Your path is yours to choose.

FAQ: Why Doesn't the NHS Routinely Test for PeriMenopause? Because your hormone levels aren't static. They fluctuate hour to hour. That's why UK doctors rely more on age, cycle changes, and symptoms than on bloodwork.

Takeaway: You're Not Lost. You're Evolving.

If it feels like your body has taken the steering wheel and driven you off-road, then breathe. This isn't a crisis. It's a recalibration. And it's the start of your return to self.

AcuWarrior™ Tip: "Two minutes a day keeps the peri away."

Because small, consistent actions like a daily acupressure ritual, a grounding breath, or an affirmation can shift everything.

Healing Breath Ritual for Everyday

Ritual steps:

1. Inhale slowly.
2. Let your breath find the places inside you that feel forgotten.
3. Exhale and say softly, "This isn't madness. It's transformation."

Affirmation

"I trust my body's rhythm. I trust myself to respond. I honour the changes as wisdom in motion, not signs of weakness."

Gratitude Prompt

Now that you've explored this chapter, take a moment to note what resonated most. Let that be your prompt: this is your time, your turning point. Find gratitude in a quiet reclaiming of your health and inner calm.

Persian Wisdom

"Every change elevates your wisdom."

هر تغییری، عقل تو را بلندتر می‌کند

Transliteration: Har taghyiri, aghl-e to ra bolandtar mikonad.

Meaning: Change isn't something to fear - it's how your body, mind, and spirit evolve. Each shift is an invitation to rise, grow, and reclaim your power.

Next Up: *We dive into symptom tracking so you can feel more in control of your body, your mind, and your PeriMenopause journey.*

CHAPTER 2

Track it to Tame it

Tracking Your Symptoms
and
Taking Charge with Clarity

Let's kick things off by getting to know your body like the back of your hand. The first step in mastering PeriMenopause is to become your own private investigator. Yes, you're about to channel your inner Miss Marple (but without the actual murder please, however tempting it may sometimes be!).

When you're in the thick of it, it might feel like everything is happening at once: mood swings, night sweats, brain fog, the works. But without tracking your symptoms, you're just guessing. And guesswork? We're not about that life.

This is where symptom tracking comes in. Think of it as logging clues. Mapping your body's patterns. Building your own case file on you. Because when you know what's going on, you can actually do something about it.

Why Tracking Your Symptoms Matters

PeriMenopause can feel like a chaotic rollercoaster.Tracking? That's you getting into the driver's seat. You'll begin to spot patterns, identify triggers, and tailor your response. Instead of reacting to chaos, you'll start recognising rhythms and that changes everything.

Take this:

→ Maybe your hot flushes are worse after wine (don't panic, rosé isn't cancelled).

→ Or your sleep goes haywire when stress builds.

→ Or you've noticed your energy crashes mid-afternoon but only on certain days.

Tracking gives you answers without the overwhelm. It shifts you from "Why is this happening?" to "Ah, I see the pattern."

How Symptoms Change Over Time

PeriMenopause isn't linear. It's unpredictable terrain. Like a hike with weather that changes every mile. What shows up early (irregular periods, rage outbursts, sore boobs) might shift into new territory (joint pain, hair thinning, itchy skin).

You're not being punished, you're being rerouted and tracking helps you prepare for those changes, not just survive them.

You become the observer, curious, calm, and ready.

Throwback: Remember When…

You used to track your period like a pro. Day 1. Ovulation. PMS. 28 days. Boom. Now? Your cycle's gone rogue. One month it's 26 days. Next month it's 62. Welcome to the chaos club!

But tracking now isn't about control. It's about awareness. And maybe, just maybe, your evening check-in includes a warm mug of Sahar's Chai™, grounding, hormone-supportive, and steeped in ritual.

And Yes, You Can Still Get Pregnant!

Let's be clear: PeriMenopause is not menopause. And it definitely does not mean infertility.

If you're sexually active and not planning to start a family, stay sharp. Your body might still be ovulating, even if your period's inconsistent. Tracking helps with that, too.

Double win.

How to Track (Without Losing the Plot) - The Hooti Method™

You don't need a spreadsheet and five colour-coded pens (Unless that brings you joy. In which case carry on). You just need a method you'll actually use. No tech required unless you want it.

Step 1: Choose Your Method

Notebook, calendar, app or just your brain and a sticky note (no shame). Keep it simple. Leave it somewhere visible. The goal is ease, not perfection. Spreadsheet lovers, we see you! Everyone else, grab a notebook and let's begin.

Step 2: What to Track

Here's your cheat sheet:

1. **Symptom(s)** - What are you feeling? (E.g. bloated, wired, moody, flushed)
2. **Severity** - From 1-10. Be honest.
3. **Triggers** - Did something spark it? Stress, sugar, sleep, social overload?
4. **Relief** - What helped? (Breathwork? A walk? Acupressure? Magnesium?)

Don't overthink it. This is your logbook. Write in your own way.

Step 3: Check-In Daily

2-5 minutes. That's it. Morning or evening. Whatever suits your flow. Make it part of your ritual. Tie it to something you already do (like brushing your teeth or sipping your tea).

Pro Tip: Leave your tracker near the kettle, your bed, or in your bag.

Step 4: Reflect Weekly

→ Once a week, pause and look at what's unfolding.

→ Are your symptoms linked to certain days?

→ Is wine or caffeine playing a role?

→ Is stress stealing your sleep?

→ Are certain remedies helping more than others?

This is your time to adjust and own your rhythm.

Your Weekly Symptom Tracker The Hooti Method™ (Example)

Date	Symptom(s)	Severity (1-10)	Possible Triggers	What Helped
3rd November	Brain fog, fatigue	7	Poor sleep, overthinking	PC6 acupressure, tea, nap
4th November	Bloating	6	Dairy, stress	Peppermint tea, walking
5th November	Anxiety, palpitations	8	Meeting overload, sugar	Breathing, rose oil

Use this as inspiration. There's no wrong way, just your way.

Quick Wins

- Choose a tracking method that works for you.
- Keep it consistent. Little notes add up.
- Reflect weekly. Patterns = power.
- Celebrate your wins and adjust gently.

Healing Breath Ritual & Affirmation

Ritual steps:

1. Close your eyes.
2. Inhale through your nose for four.
3. Hold for four.
4. Exhale through your mouth for six.
5. Repeat softly: "I trust the signals. I honour the rhythms. I am learning, not losing."

Gratitude Prompt

How did your body feel this week? What's one small win you noticed - and one gentle shift you can carry into next week?

Set a timer. Brew your tea. Give yourself five quiet minutes.

This isn't a chore. It's care.

Persian Wisdom

"Every moment is a new moment."

هر لحظه، لحظه‌ی نو است

Transliteration: Har lahzeh, lahzeh-ye no ast.

Meaning: No matter what just happened, you can begin again - right now. PeriMenopause reminds us to honour each moment as a fresh start.

You are not behind. You are right on time.

***Let's Keep Talking**: Tag me using* **#PocketPeri** *and mention @AcuCareClinicUK. I'd love to know how this chapter has helped you.*

***Next Up:** We move from the notepad to the body and explore how Advanced Acupressure and Aromatherapy can support your nervous system, your hormones and your sense of self.*

CHAPTER 3

The Foundations

Simple Tools for Real Relief

Before we dive into specific symptoms like hot flushes, mood swings, or skin changes, let's lay a little groundwork. This chapter is your personal starter kit introducing three essential tools that will appear again and again throughout the book:

- The Press-Pulsate-Pause Method™ for quick physical relief.
- Healing Breath Rituals to reset your nervous system.
- Aromatherapy for PeriMenopause Support, grounded in both ancient and clinical wisdom.

You don't have to master everything at once. These tools are here to be picked up, tested, and returned to whenever needed. Think of this chapter as your backstage pass to your body's inner rhythm and your right to feel better.

AcuWarrior™ Tip: Search for the QR code in each chapter to get help with Advanced Acupressure point locations.

The Press-Pulsate-Pause Method™

Press - Pulsate - Pause.

Welcome to your go-to Advanced Acupressure (i.e acupuncture without needles) technique. You'll see each acupressure point's Chinese name in brackets).

Whether you're feeling overwhelmed, wired, foggy, or flat, this method taps into your body's innate intelligence to reset and rebalance.

Here's how it works:

Use calm, measured, breathing for each step.

Press - Find the suggested acupressure point (each chapter will guide you). Press firmly for 30-60 seconds. This stimulates nerve endings and signals your brain to release endorphins (your natural stress-relieving, pain-reducing, chemicals).

Pulsate - Rather than holding the pressure still, begin a gentle pulse - pressing and releasing in a rhythm. This boosts circulation, helps shift stagnation (a key idea in Chinese medicine), and enhances therapeutic results.

Pause - Let go and rest for 30 seconds. This gives your body a moment to respond, settle, and integrate the effect. This step is often overlooked but this is where the deeper healing begins.

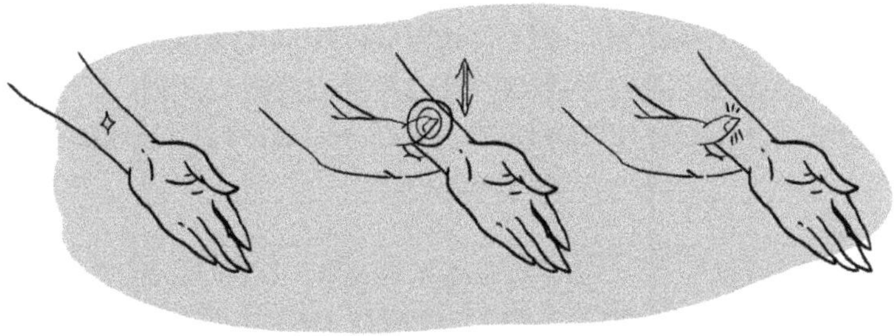

You can repeat the sequence on the same point or move to another, depending on your symptoms. This technique takes just 2-3 minutes and can be used anytime, anywhere. Daily routines are recommended for best results.

AcuWarrior™ Reminder:

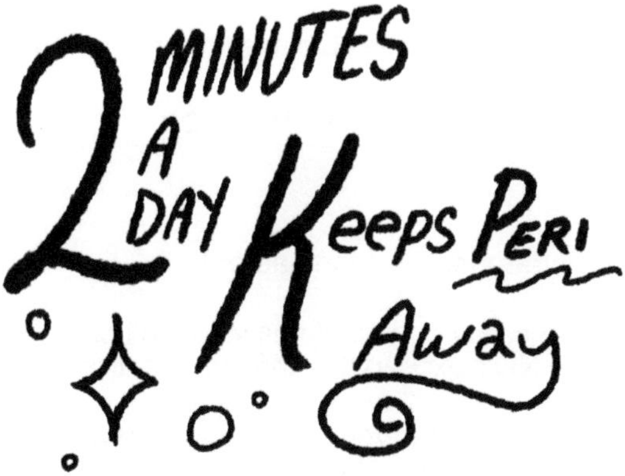

You'll see the Press-Pulsate-Pause Method™ referenced in later chapters. Look out for QR codes to access video demonstrations.

Safety Note: The Press-Pulsate-Pause Method™ should not be performed on an empty stomach or when you are too full. Don't worry if you struggle to find the precise point location because the beauty of advanced acupressure is that as long as you're in the vicinity and apply the correct technique you can't miss it.

Aromatherapy for PeriMenopause Support

Safe. Grounded. Personal.

Essential oils are everywhere but not all advice is created equal. The truth?

- Not all oils are hormone-safe.
- Not all application methods are suitable.
- And, sadly, not everyone offering aromatherapy is trained.

Just because it's "natural" doesn't mean it's harmless.

I trained in aromatherapy alongside beauty therapy sciences and have used it clinically for years, blending this skill with Traditional Chinese Medicine diagnosis to craft bespoke remedies for my patients. I don't just throw oils together. I assess each client's root imbalance (Liver stagnation? Spleen deficiency? Kidney depletion?) and build a tailored blend from there. That's why in this book, you won't find "DIY recipes." I don't know your full health picture and I'd never recommend guesswork when it comes to your hormones.

Instead, here's a safe, accessible, way to get started:

Damp Cotton Wool Aromatherapy

How to use it:

1. Lightly dampen a cotton pad or ball.
2. Add 1-2 drops of a single essential oil or a combination of oils but DO NOT exceed the safe limit of drops.
3. Hold the pad near your nostrils and take slow, deep, breaths in through your nose. Breathe out gently through your mouth, continuing for at least 30 seconds to a minute.
4. Then place it near you, on your desk, bedside table, on your chest over clothing, secured to your wrist with a hairband, or even tucked into your bra (making sure there is no direct skin contact).

The water slows down evaporation and reduces intensity making it a gentle, effective, low-risk way to enjoy the benefits.

Safe starter oils:

- Lavender for sleep, tension, or anxiety.
- Sweet orange for heaviness and low mood.
- Clary sage for hormonal fatigue (avoid in pregnancy).
- Geranium for emotional swings and circulation.

AromaAcu Therapy™

This is when the healing powers of Aromatherapy meet with the Press-Pulsate-Pause Method™ and are applied simultaneously. Here, you've got a powerful healing combo which I use in my clinic and it works wonders at home too. It's my signature approach to support both body and mind.

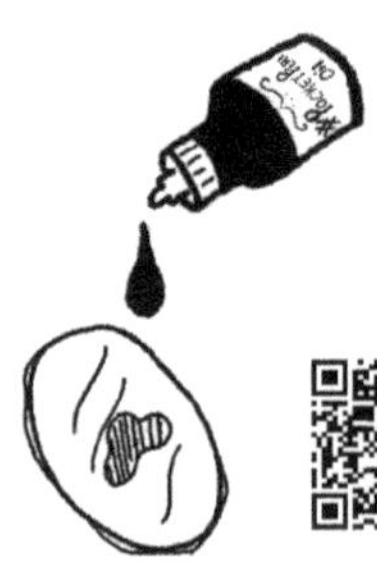

How to: Start by holding the pad close to your nostrils and taking slow, deep, breaths in through your nose, gently exhaling through your mouth for 30 seconds to a minute. Then, place the pad somewhere such as your wrist, desk, or clothing and carry out the Press-Pulsate-Pause Method™ on your chosen Advanced Acupressure point.

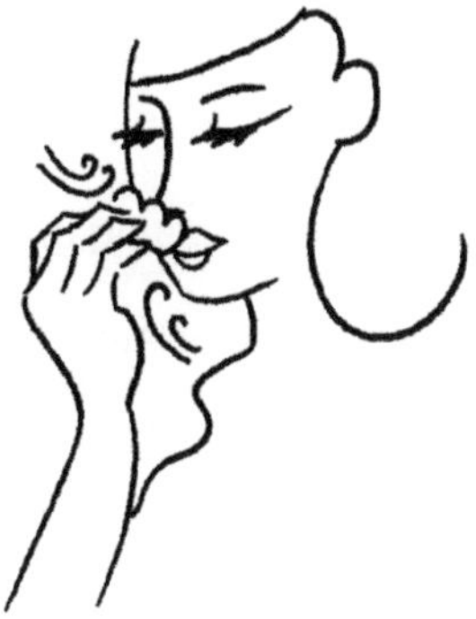

Safety Note: Always keep essential oils away from children and pets, especially cats and dogs. While I truly believe applying diluted, prescription oil blends to the skin can be helpful in the right context, I don't recommend self-prescribing. Sometimes what works for one person won't suit another. Never apply neat essential oils to skin unless trained. Being empowered doesn't mean going rogue.It means knowing your tools and your limits. If you'd like personalised guidance, seek a qualified aromatherapist, or you're welcome to book an online consultation with me. I support patients worldwide.

Healing Breath Rituals

Little moments. Big impact.

These aren't your average breathing exercises. They're subtle, sacred tools that reconnect you with the organs most affected during PeriMenopause - your liver, spleen, heart, kidneys and more.

Rooted in my clinical practice, these rituals help you:

- Regulate emotions.
- Soothe an overactive nervous system.
- Reclaim space in your own body.

You'll be gently introduced to these organ-based rituals in later chapters.

When you see the breath symbol, that's your cue to pause, close your eyes, and come back to yourself.

I've paired these rituals with Mantra's and/or Affirmations to use alongside. Take your pick!

This isn't about escaping your body. It's about coming home to it.

Why This Chapter Matters

This is your anchor. Your body is changing but you're not powerless.

These three tools (the Press-Pulsate-Pause Method™, Healing Breath Rituals, and Aromatherapy wisdom) will continue to support you throughout this journey. They're free, natural, and yours.

The more you use them, the more your body will respond. Not overnight but over time, consistently.

Please note: As you explore each chapter, you may notice certain acupressure points and essential oils appearing more than once. That's no coincidence. Each point and oil has multiple therapeutic functions, and when used with different intentions or combinations, they support the body in unique ways. That's the beauty of holistic healing: versatile, powerful, and deeply intuitive.

Quick Wins

- The Press-Pulsate-Pause Method™. Use it throughout this book for acupressure-based symptom relief.
- Healing Breath Rituals. Gentle breathwork tools that connect you to your internal rhythms.
- Safe Aromatherapy. A calm, low-risk way to support mood and hormones, one drop at a time.

Affirmation

"I honour the quiet wisdom within. With every breath, every pause, and every press of my fingertips, I return to balance, one moment at a time."

Gratitude Prompt

Which tool spoke to you most? The Press-Pulsate-Pause Method™, the Healing Breath Ritual, or Aromatherapy?

Write down one moment this week where you paused, breathed, or tried something new.

That's your win. That's your shift. You're not behind, you've just begun.

Persian Wisdom

"Relief begins when you return to yourself."

آرامش وقتی می‌آید که به خودت بازگردی

Transliteration: Ârâmesh vaghti miâyad ke be khodet bâzgardi.

Meaning: You don't need to search far and wide. The answers (your breath, your body, your wisdom) are already within you.

***Let's Keep Talking**: Tag me using* **#PocketPeri** *and mention @AcuCareClinicUK. I'd love to know your thoughts on these healing methods.*

***Next Up**: We look at hormones and the basics of PeriMenopause. You're not chasing balance. You're building it, one breath, one press, one moment at a time.*

CHAPTER 4

Hormones and You

Understanding the Basics of PeriMenopause

You're not going crazy, and, no, it's not just stress. What you're feeling, whether it's mood swings, hot flushes, or fatigue, isn't "all in your head." It's your hormones my darling and they've been quietly running the show in the background for decades.

Now they're shifting. And with that shift, everything from your sleep to your skin may feel offbeat. But here's the good news! Understanding what's happening inside your body is your superpower.

Let's decode the science and honour the ancient medicine that's been explaining this transition long before the word "PeriMenopause" existed.

What Are Hormones, Anyway?

Hormones are your body's internal messengers sending chemical signals zipping around your bloodstream, telling tissues and organs what to do. They influence everything from your metabolism to your mood and menstrual cycle.

During PeriMenopause, those messengers start whispering instead of shouting. The communication becomes less clear, more erratic, and that's when symptoms start to show.

Let's look at the big players:

- **Oestrogen** - The Queen Bee. Responsible for your cycle, skin glow, brain sharpness, and even joint lubrication. As levels drop, cue hot flushes, brain fog, and mood swings.

- **Progesterone** - The natural calm-down hormone. It helps you sleep, stabilises mood, and keeps oestrogen in check. When it dips, expect more anxiety, irritability, and restless nights.

- **Testosterone** - Often overlooked, but key to libido, drive, and muscle tone. Its gradual decline can leave you feeling flat, unmotivated, or disconnected from your sensual self.

The Hormonal Cascade of PeriMenopause

Think of it like a hormonal game of Jenga. Pull out one block and the whole tower wobbles. It's rarely just one hormone in isolation and it's the imbalance between them that causes chaos.

- Oestrogen dips → Thermostat issues (hot flushes), mood changes, vaginal dryness.

- Progesterone declines → Anxiety, sleep disruption, shorter or irregular cycles.

- Testosterone falls → Energy slumps, lower libido, muscle weakness.

This isn't a malfunction. It's a recalibration and while it may feel disorienting, it's possible to navigate this with more ease, once you understand what's going on.

Western Science Meets Ancient Wisdom: A TCM Perspective

In Traditional Chinese Medicine (TCM), PeriMenopause is seen as a natural energetic shift, not a disorder. The body is adjusting from a state of fertility to a new internal rhythm and it's all rooted in the Kidneys.

Not to be confused with the anatomical kidneys alone, the Kidney system in TCM governs:

- Hormonal balance.
- Brain function and memory.
- Bone strength and aging.
- Reproductive health.

It's known as the "Root of Life" and the reservoir of your vitality and genetic blueprint. What's fascinating is that modern science is catching up. Research shows a strong link between brain function, hormonal shifts, and the hypothalamic-pituitary-ovarian (HPO) axis which mirrors the Kidney system's role in regulating neuroendocrine balance.

Modern scans like functional MRIs (fMRIs) confirm that hormone fluctuations directly influence regions of the brain linked to mood, memory, and temperature regulation, validating what TCM has been saying for thousands of years. So while your blood test might look "normal", TCM helps us make sense of the senseless, especially when conventional medicine leaves you feeling dismissed.

How Hormonal Shifts Affect Your Body

Let's break it down symptom by symptom and look at what's going on underneath:

- **Brain Fog**: Oestrogen supports neurotransmitter activity and blood flow to the brain. When it drops, so does your clarity and recall. It's not just forgetfulness, it's biochemical.
- **Hot Flushes & Night Sweats**: Your internal thermostat goes haywire. The hypothalamus (the body's heat regulator) becomes more sensitive to subtle shifts. This is a direct result of lower oestrogen.
- **Mood Swings**: Less progesterone = less GABA activity (your brain's calming neurotransmitter). Add in fluctuating oestrogen

and you've got an emotional rollercoaster.

- **Libido Drop**: Testosterone fuels desire and pleasure response. Its decline, combined with stress and sleep loss, can quieten your sex drive.

- **Sleep Disruption**: Oestrogen supports melatonin and serotonin regulation. Without it, your circadian rhythm suffers and so do your nights.

How to Support Your Hormones During PeriMenopause

This isn't about doing everything. It's about doing the right things consistently, gently, and wisely.

The Press-Pulsate-Pause Method™ for General Use

You read about this in Chapter 3 and now's the time to apply it.

- **Kidney 3 太溪 (Tài Xī)**
    - Inside ankle, between the Achilles tendon and ankle bone.
    - Supports hormonal balance and brain health.

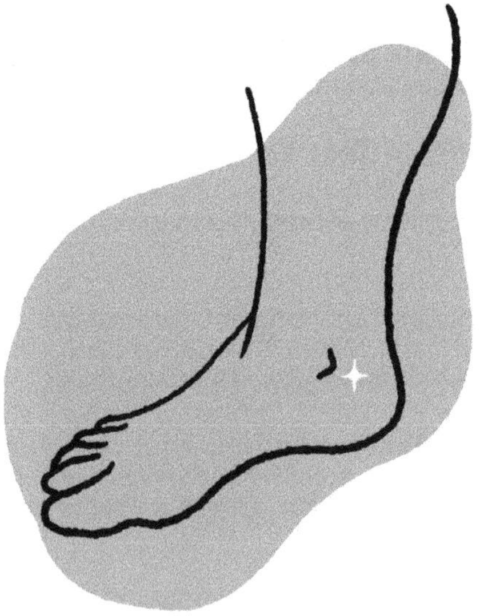

- **Liver 3 太衝 (Tài Chōng)**
    - Top of foot, between the first and second toes.
    - Great for stress, emotional flow, and menstrual regulation.

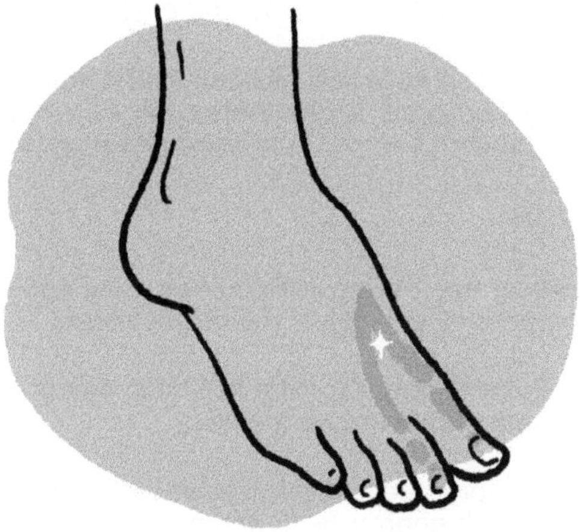

Please Note: You can use as many points as you need, as long as you feel grounded and well-fed. Avoid using pressure if you're feeling faint, extremely hungry, or unwell. Start with 1-2 points, and build as your body responds.

AcuWarrior™ Reminder: "Two minutes a day keeps the peri away."

AromaAcu Therapy™ for Hormonal Support

We covered the safety principles in Chapter 3 so here's how to practise them now.

- Dampen cotton wool.
- Add 1-2 total drops of essential oil (never more).
- Place nearby (desk, pillow, bra- avoid skin contact).

You can repeat this up to 2-3 times a day.

Recommended oils:

- Clary Sage - Supports oestrogen balance and mood (avoid during pregnancy).
- Lavender - Calms the nervous system, improves sleep.
- Geranium - Aids circulation and hormonal regulation.
- Sweet Orange - Lifts low mood and emotional heaviness.

Less is more. Overuse of essential oils can overstimulate or sensitise your system. In my own clinic, aromatherapy is always guided by diagnosis with no random blends. Your body deserves the same respect.

Diet & Nutrition

- **Phytoestrogens**: Found in flaxseeds, tofu, and lentils, these plant compounds can lightly mimic oestrogen.
- **Healthy Fats**: Omega-3s from fish, chia seeds, and walnuts support brain and hormone function.
- **Hydration**: Hormonal shifts increase water loss. Aim for 2 litres a day to help with energy, skin, and mental clarity.

Healing Breath Ritual for the Kidneys

This ritual helps you tap into the foundation of your energy system, especially during low-energy or emotionally vulnerable moments.

Ritual Steps:

1. Place your hands over your lower back (above your waist).
2. Inhale deeply, visualising the breath reaching your kidneys.
3. Exhale slowly, imagining calm and stability flowing into the area.
4. Whisper a quiet “thank you” to your kidneys for carrying you through.

Use this breath when you feel exhausted, overwhelmed, or mentally scattered. It’s subtle, yet powerful.

Quick Wins

- Your hormones are shifting but that doesn't mean you're broken.
- TCM offers a refreshingly human lens when nothing else makes sense.
- Use the tools in Chapter 3 to support your body: acupressure, aromatherapy, breath rituals.
- Less is more. Choose one thing and do it well.
- You're not chasing balance. You're building it - one breath, one press, one choice at a time.

Affirmation

"I am the boss of my hormones, steering the ship with grace and guts. Hormones don't control me. I control them."

Say it out loud. Say it again. Then say it like you mean it.

Gratitude Prompt

What are you grateful for today?

Write down one thing, no matter how small. Gratitude rewires your brain and your hormones respond.

Persian Wisdom

"Even the moon has phases. So do you."

ماه هم دور دارد، زن هم چنین است

Transliteration: Mâh ham dowr dârad, zan ham chenin ast.

Meaning: Just like nature, your cycles are sacred. Hormones rise and fall, not as flaws, but as part of your design.

***Let's Keep Talking**: Tag me using **#PocketPeri** and mention @AcuCareClinicUK - I'd love to know which tool you tried first.*

***Next Up**: The PeriMenopause brain (you know this has been on your mind for a while). Did you know the symptoms of PeriMenopause can last up to 8 years (that's nearly a decade of your life). No wonder your brain is screaming for support.*

CHAPTER 5

The PeriMenopause Brain

Staying Sharp and Understanding the Cognitive Changes

One minute you're mid-conversation, the next you're blanking on someone's name and it's someone you've known for years. Welcome to brain fog, one of the most irritating (and surprisingly common) symptoms of PeriMenopause.

It's not all hot flushes and night sweats. For many women, PeriMenopause starts in the mind with memory glitches, focus fumbles, and that unsettling sense that your brain has taken a temporary holiday.

You're not losing your mind, but your brain is going through a shift. And once you understand why, you can work with it and not against it.

What's Going On In Your Brain?

Oestrogen and progesterone aren't just about periods and pregnancy. They're also brain fuel. These hormones support neurotransmitters (chemical messengers that regulate memory, mood, and mental sharpness), and they influence blood flow, inflammation, and even how your brain uses glucose for energy. So when those hormones start fluctuating, the result is less clarity and more fog.

According to neuroscientist Dr Lisa Mosconi, the brain undergoes measurable metabolic changes during PeriMenopause. That's why you might notice that you:

- Have trouble finding words mid-sentence.
- Are forgetting names, dates, or appointments.
- Have difficulty concentrating or making decisions.
- Experience emotional overwhelm.

The good news? These changes aren't permanent. With the right support, your brain can recalibrate and even thrive.

A TCM Perspective: The Brain-Kidney Connection

Traditional Chinese Medicine has long recognised what science is only now confirming, that shifts in hormones affect the brain. In TCM, the Kidney system is seen as the "Root of Life." but it doesn't just govern fertility. It also stores your vital essence, supports brain function, and influences aging. In fact, in ancient texts, the Kidneys were directly linked to brain health.

Modern science now agrees with functional MRI scans (fMRI) showing clear links between the hypothalamic-pituitary-ovarian (HPO) axis and the parts of the brain that regulate memory, mood, and cognition.

When we support the Kidneys (from a TCM view), we're not just working with hormones. We're nourishing the brain both physically and emotionally.

The Press-Pulsate-Pause Method™ for Brain Health

(Refer to Chapter 3 for full instructions)

Your daily acupressure reset is right at your fingertips. These Advanced Acupressure points stimulate the nervous system and boost blood flow to the brain, giving you a sense of clarity, calm, and control.

- **Third Eye 印堂 (Yìn Táng)**
    - Between the eyebrows.
    - Known to calm the mind, relieve tension, and sharpen focus.

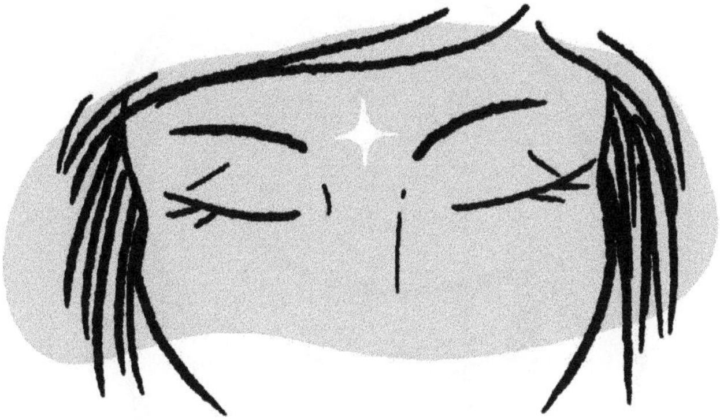

- **Kidney 1 涌泉 (Yǒng Quán)**
    - Found on the sole of the foot, about one-third of the way down from the base of the toes towards the heel, in the soft dip between the ball of the foot and the arch - roughly in line with the second and third toes.
    - Helps ground scattered energy and supports brain-Kidney balance.

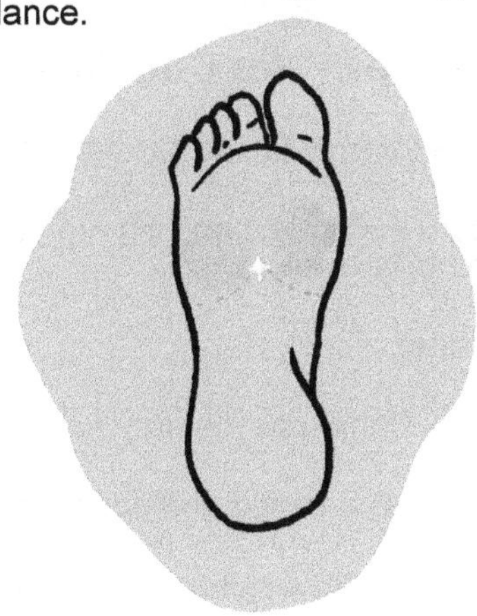

- **DU20 百会 (Bǎi Huì)**
    - Crown of the head in line with the tips of your ears.
    - Lifts energy, brightens mood, and supports mental sharpness.

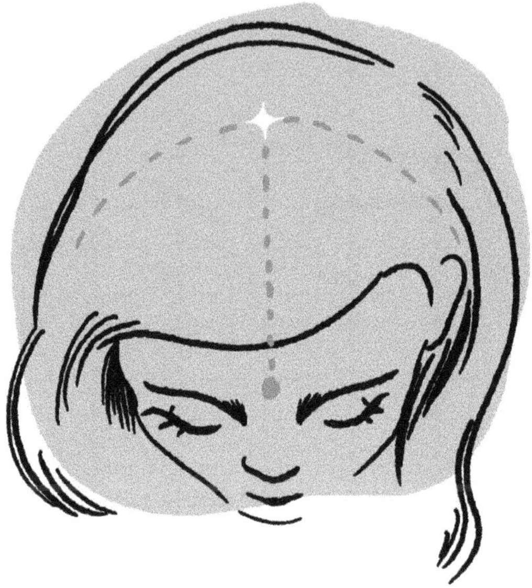

AcuWarrior™ Reminder: "Two minutes a day keeps the peri away."

This is your reset button. Use it daily. Breathe, press, and come back to yourself.

AromaAcu Therapy™ for Cognitive Calm

(Refer to Chapter 3 for how to use oils safely)

This is my signature method combining aromatherapy with Advanced Acupressure to amplify results.

Recommended oils:

- Rosemary - Enhances memory and alertness.
- Peppermint - Clears fog and boosts focus.
- Lavender - Reduces stress and overthinking.

Supplements That Support the Brain

Food is always your foundation but certain supplements may help give your brain a boost during this phase.

Top Supportive Nutrients:

- Magnesium L-Threonate - A highly absorbable form shown to support cognitive performance.
- Omega-3 (DHA + EPA) - Essential for memory and mood.
- Vitamin D3 - Low levels are linked to cognitive decline and low mood.

See your health professional or you're welcome to book a consultation with me. I can recommend trusted brands that I use with my own patients.

Quick Wins

1. Daily Press-Pulsate-Pause Method™ - use acupressure to stimulate your brain.
2. Add AromaAcu Therapy™ - especially in the morning or before a busy day.
3. Support with supplements - after seeking professional advice.
4. Breathe! The Healing Breath Ritual brings it all together.
5. Combine the "Press-Pulsate-Pause Method™, breathwork, with consistency.

Healing Breath Ritual for Mental Clarity & Calm

Ritual steps:

1. Place both hands over your forehead.
2. Inhale deeply through your nose, visualising cool air flowing into your brain.
3. Exhale slowly through your mouth, imagining a wave of light clearing mental clutter.
4. Whisper softly: "Thank you, mind. I see you."

Use this when you feel mentally foggy, forgetful, or overwhelmed. It's subtle yet powerful.

Affirmation

"I feed my mind with clarity, calm, and confidence. My brain is my power centre, and I nurture it to stay focused and fabulous."

Gratitude Prompt

Your brain is not broken, it's just rewiring. This week, pause and ask yourself: What's one thing my brain still does brilliantly, even on the foggy days? When did I surprise myself with clarity, intuition, or creativity?

Jot it down. Celebrate it. Your mind is adapting, not disappearing. Let this be your reminder: there's strength in the shift.

Persian Wisdom

"The mind is a garden, water it with calm."

ذهن باغی‌ست، با آرامش آبیاری‌اش کن

Transliteration: Zehn bâghi-st, bâ ârâmesh âbyâri-ash kon.

Meaning: A foggy mind isn't failure. It's a call to pause, nourish, and come back clearer. Let calm be your clarity.

Let's Keep Talking*: Tag me using* **#PocketPeri** *and mention @AcuCareClinicUK. I'd love to see what works for your brain.*

Next Up*: Mood swings and emotional balance. Yes, we're going there. The mind and emotions are linked and we're exploring how to reclaim your mood, regulate emotions, and ride the rollercoaster with a little more grace for yourself.*

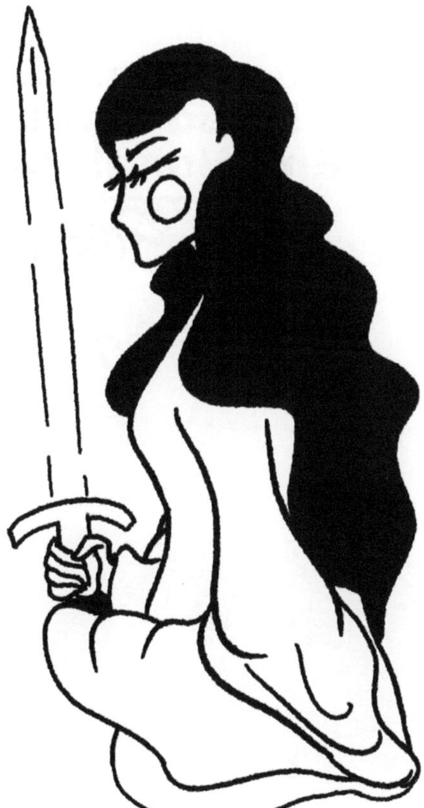

CHAPTER 6

Mood Swings & Emotional Balance

Ah, the joy of PeriMenopause. One minute you're on top of the world, the next you're crying over cold tea or snapping at someone who breathed too loudly.

Sound familiar? You're not alone. This chapter is your emotional survival kit, blending Advanced Acupressure, Aromatherapy, breathwork and science-backed self-awareness to help you feel better, not just function.

Because here's the truth: It's not just "in your head." It's in your hormones.

Why Mood Swings Happen (And Why It's Not Your Fault)

Your hormones (particularly oestrogen and progesterone) don't just control your cycle. They also influence your neurotransmitters (chemical messengers in your brain that affect mood, focus, and calm).

- Oestrogen helps boost serotonin, the brain's natural stabiliser. When oestrogen drops, your emotional buffer drops too.
- Progesterone is your natural relaxant. When it fluctuates or drops, anxiety, irritation, and restlessness often follow.

You're not overreacting.You're recalibrating - chemically, biologically, and emotionally.

TCM Insight: The Organ-Emotion Connection

In Traditional Chinese Medicine, emotional imbalance isn't just "emotional", it's physiological.

Each emotion is tied to an organ system:

- **Liver** - Linked to stress, frustration, and repressed anger. When Liver energy becomes stagnant, it can lead to outbursts or feelings of being "on edge."
- **Heart** - Home of the Shen (your spirit and emotional consciousness). When the Heart is disturbed, it can show up as anxiety, panic, or scattered thoughts.
- **Spleen** - Governs worry and overthinking. When depleted, it makes you feel foggy, drained, and mentally stuck.

When hormones shift (like during PeriMenopause) these organ systems become more sensitive. The result? Emotions that feel overwhelming, out of character, or hard to shake, but here's the empowering part. When you support these systems, you support your emotional landscape too. That's why this chapter's rituals work. They aren't just soothing, they're recalibrating.

Let's Talk About the Rage

It's one of the most misunderstood symptoms of PeriMenopause and one of the most common. That explosive, out-of-nowhere fury that makes you feel like a stranger in your own skin?

It's not your personality, it's your biology.

When oestrogen dips, serotonin can crash, and suddenly, the tiniest thing (crumbs on the counter, a slow reply, the wrong look) can feel unbearable.

You're not "too emotional." You're hormonally overwhelmed. And you deserve support, not shame. We'll go even deeper into emotional imbalances, like stress, anxiety, and worry in the next chapter.

The Press-Pulsate-Pause Method™ for Emotional Balance

(Refer to Chapter 3 for full instructions)

Welcome to your 2-minute Daily Ritual. Use this Advanced Acupressure Point Combination to regulate mood, calm the nervous system, and reconnect with your emotional core without spiralling.

- **Heart 7 神门 (Shén Mén)**
    - Inner wrist crease, in line with your little finger.
    - Calms anxiety and helps settle emotional overwhelm.

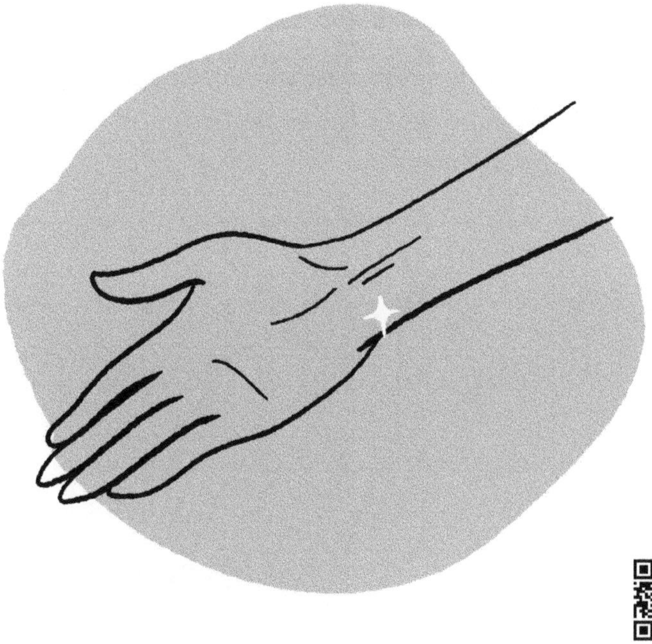

- **Third Eye 印堂 (Yìn Táng)**
    - Between the eyebrows.
    - Soothes the mind and supports restful focus.

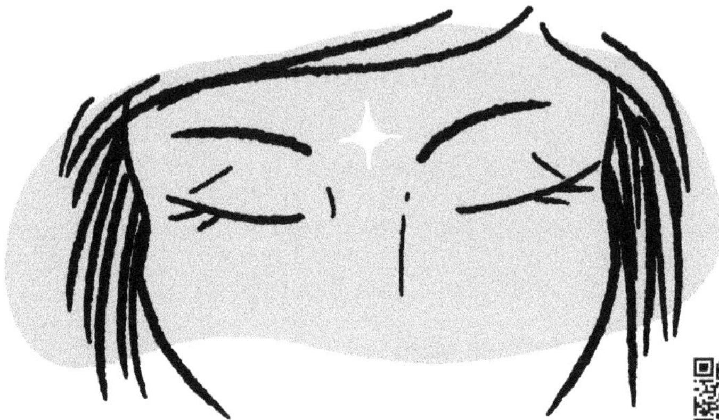

- **Large Intestine 4 合谷 (Hé Gǔ)**
    - Between thumb and index finger.
    - Supports stress relief and mood regulation via the vagus nerve.
    - Avoid if pregnant.

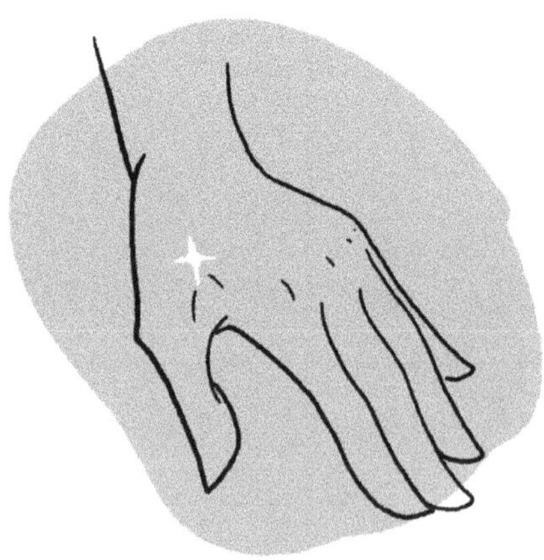

AcuWarrior™ Reminder: "Two minutes a day keeps the peri away."

AromaAcu Therapy™ for Natural Mood Medicine

(Refer to Chapter 3 for how to use oils safely)

Essential oils influence the brain's limbic system, which governs mood, memory, and emotional responses. Inhaling the right oils at the right time can help regulate stress, soothe anxiety, and shift emotional states.

Recommended oils:

- Lavender - Calms anxiety, helps you breathe deeper, and unwinds internal tension.
- Rose - Soothes emotional intensity and supports serotonin.
- Peppermint - Clears mental fog and cools heated emotions.

Internal Support for a Steadier Mood

Sometimes, even with the best self-care rituals, your nervous system needs a little more backup.

Supplements like:

- Magnesium Glycinate - Known for its calming effect on the nervous system.
- Vitamin B6 - Supports hormone balance and neurotransmitter production (your brain's messengers).
- L-Theanine - Helps ease anxiety and promote a sense of calm.

Supplements can gently support mood regulation, especially during hormonal shifts. But it's not one-size-fits-all. Always check with your healthcare provider before adding supplements, especially if you're taking medication for mood, anxiety, or depression. You're also welcome to book a supplement consultation with me if you'd like a more tailored approach.

Healing Breath Ritual for Emotional Release

This calming breathwork technique helps release emotional tension without suppressing it.

Ritual steps:

1. Sit with feet grounded, hands on your belly.
2. Inhale through your nose for 4 counts.
3. Hold for 2 counts and observe the emotion without judgement.
4. Exhale for 6 counts through the mouth and release what's no longer serving you.
5. Repeat for 5-10 cycles.

Each breath is a quiet protest against burnout, and a powerful reclaiming of peace.

Quick Wins

- Press-Pulsate-Pause Method™ - Use Heart 7 or Yin Tang.
- Aromatherapy - Inhale lavender or rose using the Damp Cotton Wool Method.
- Healing Breath Ritual - Let go of the pressure to hold it all together.
- Supplement Support - Nutrient gaps can worsen emotional instability.
- See your health professional or you're welcome to book a supplement consultation with me.

Affirmation

"I allow my emotions to move through me, not define me. I trust myself to return to calm."

Gratitude Prompt

Your emotions aren't the enemy. They're messengers. This week, ask yourself what emotion showed up loudest and what was it trying to tell me? Instead of judging it, how can I thank it for showing me what I need?

Mood swings don't mean you're broken.They mean your body is asking to be heard and you need to listen. Let this reflection be your moment of grace.

Persian Wisdom

"Relief begins when you return to yourself."

آرامش وقتی می‌آید که به خودت بازگردی

Transliteration: Ârâmesh vaghti miâyad ke be khodet bâzgardi.

Meaning: You don't need to search far and wide. The answers - your breath, your body, your wisdom - are already within you.

Let's Keep Talking: *Tag @AcuCareClinicUK and use* **#PocketPeri**. *I'd love to know what works for your emotional flow.*

Next Up: *We go deeper into the fog, the fatigue, and the flatness that no one warned you about. It's time to give your nervous system the reset it's been begging for.*

CHAPTER 7

Beyond Mood Swings

The Deep Emotional Reset

Experiencing stress, anxiety, fear, grief, or burnout? This chapter gives your nervous system what it actually needs.

One minute you're managing life just fine. The next, your chest is tight, your mind is spiralling, or you burst into tears over something as minor as the wrong parking space. Welcome to the deeper emotional landscape of PeriMenopause. The one that goes far beyond mood swings. It's not just about feeling irritable. It's the emotional weight of invisible pressure: the panic, the fear, the not-enoughness. The "I can't do this anymore." And here's the thing: you're not overreacting. Your nervous system is overwhelmed.

Hormones don't just regulate periods. They modulate stress responses, neurotransmitters (your brain's chemical messengers), and how your body handles pressure. When oestrogen declines, cortisol sensitivity spikes. Your body feels stress more acutely, and your emotional resilience can feel like it's eroding.

But that doesn't mean you're powerless. This chapter is your reset. Let's start by understanding what's really happening.

What Stress Really Does During PeriMenopause

From a Western perspective:

- Cortisol (your main stress hormone) becomes harder to regulate when oestrogen drops. You may feel wired but tired, anxious, or hyper-alert.
- GABA and serotonin (your calming neurotransmitters) also decline with falling oestrogen - which explains the creeping anxiety, broken sleep, and emotional volatility.
- Chronic stress contributes to inflammation, fatigue, and even weight gain - not laziness, not ageing, not "just life."

From a TCM perspective:

- The Liver becomes overloaded, leading to emotional suppression, irritability, and internal tension.
- The Kidneys, which store your Jing (deep vitality), become depleted under chronic stress and fear.
- The Heart, which houses the Shen (spirit), becomes unsettled, causing panic, racing thoughts, and insomnia.

Translation? You're not broken but your inner systems are asking for backup.

The Press-Pulsate-Pause Method™ for Emotional Overload

(Refer to Chapter 3 for full instructions)

These are the points I use in-clinic when patients feel emotionally fried. Do one, two, or all. Whatever suits your day.

- **Kidney 1 涌泉 (Yǒng Quán)**
  - Found on the sole of the foot, about one-third of the way down from the base of the toes towards the heel, in the soft dip between the ball of the foot and the arch - roughly in line with the second and third toes.
  - Anchors fear, calms the nervous system, and gently resets your fight-or-flight state.

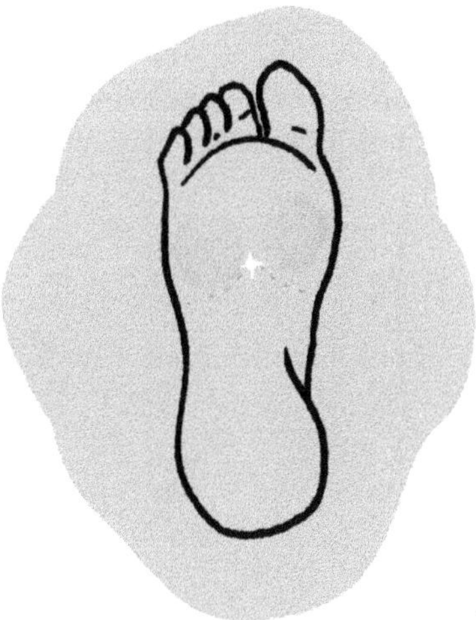

AcuWarrior™ Tip: Do this when you feel overwhelmed or frozen.

- **Pericardium 6 内关 (Nèi Guān)**
    - Three finger-widths below the wrist on the inner arm.
    - Calms the Heart, soothes nausea, and steadies the mind. For those moments when you can't switch off.

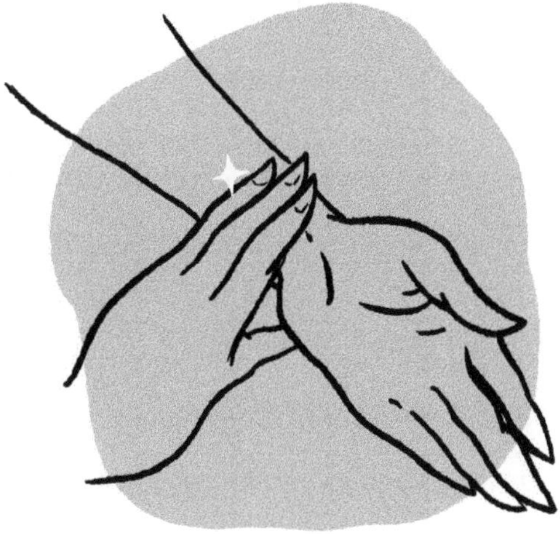

- **Liver 3 太冲 (Tài Chōng)**
    - Top of the foot, between the first and second toe bones.
    - Supports emotional release and helps regulate tension, irritability, and internalised stress. Bye bye snappy snaps!

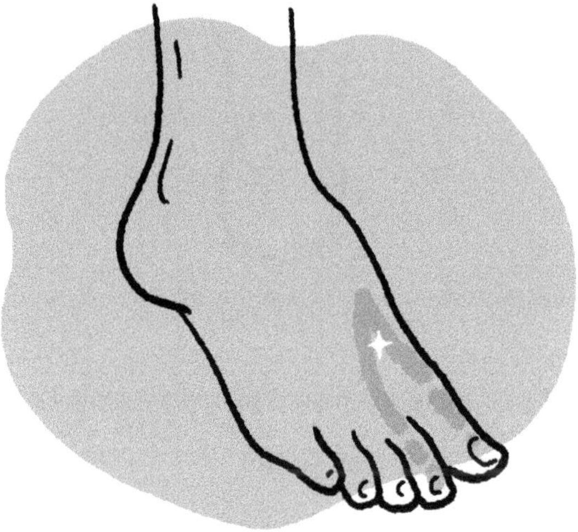

AcuWarrior™ Reminder: "Two minutes a day keeps the peri away." Build this into your daily reset. Your nervous system will thank you.

AromaAcu Therapy™ for the Overstimulated Mind

(Refer to Chapter 3 for how to use oils safely)

Choose one oil depending on how you feel. Then pair it with the point that speaks to you. This is nervous system care, reimagined.

- Chamomile - Gently soothes anxiety and inner restlessness. Use with PC6.
- Vetiver - Grounds the body and mind.
- Rose - Eases grief and emotional heartache.
- Bergamot - Uplifts and relieves low mood or burnout.

Supplements That May Help (But Check First)

When stress hijacks your body, it depletes minerals and disrupts neurotransmitters. Some supplements can help, but always check with your health professional (especially if you're on meds for anxiety, sleep, or mood):

- Magnesium glycinate - Calms the nervous system without causing drowsiness.
- L-theanine - Supports calm alertness and balances brain waves.
- Ashwagandha - An adaptogen that may help reduce cortisol levels.
- B-complex - Supports energy and helps regulate stress responses.

See your health professional or you're welcome to book a supplement consultation with me.

Healing Breath Ritual For Emotional Reset

Use this when your chest feels tight, your mind is racing, or your emotions feel too big.

Ritual steps:

- Place one hand on your chest, the other on your lower belly.
- Inhale slowly through your nose for 4 seconds. Feel both hands rise.
- Hold your breath for 4 seconds.
- Exhale through your mouth for 6-8 seconds, imagining stress leaving your body.
- Repeat for 2-3 minutes. Whisper this if it helps: "I am safe, I am here, I am enough."

Quick Wins

- Drink water - Even mild dehydration worsens stress.
- Move your body - Just 10 minutes of walking helps.
- Snack smart - Dips in blood sugar can amplify emotional chaos.
- Silence the noise - Turn off notifications, even if just for 20 minutes.

Gratitude Prompt

This isn't weakness, it's a signal.Your body is trying to protect you. Your emotions are asking for care, not critique.

This week ask yourself what moment made me feel overwhelmed and how did I respond? What helped soothe my nervous system, even briefly?

Write it down. Breathe into it.Then thank yourself, not for being "strong," but for staying present. That's the real power.

Persian Wisdom

"Grief is the price we pay for love. But the soul learns to breathe again."

غم بهای دوست داشتن است، اما جان دوباره نفس می‌کشد

Transliteration: Gham bahāye doost dāshtan ast, ammā jān dobāre nafas mikeshe.

Meaning: Emotions can shake us, but they don't destroy us. Even in grief or burnout, the soul can return to calm. Don't silence what you feel, just find a gentler way to hold it.

Let's Keep Talking: *Tag me using* **#PocketPeri** *and mention @AcuCareClinicUK - let me know how this chapter landed for you.*

Next Up: *We talk about heart health. It's time to reconnect with the rhythm of your body. Palpitations, panic, heartbreak - we're going there.*

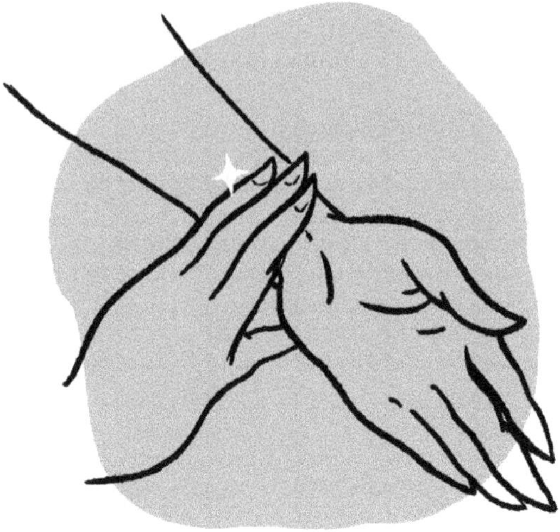

- **Lung 7 列缺 (Liè Quē)**
    - Located on the thumb side of your wrist, about one and a half finger widths above the wrist crease. You'll find it in a slight dip, just off to the side of the bone. It's often easier to feel when your palm is turned towards you.
    - Opens the chest, clears emotional grief, and helps manage sweating. Eases breathlessness, being teary, or sweating from stress.

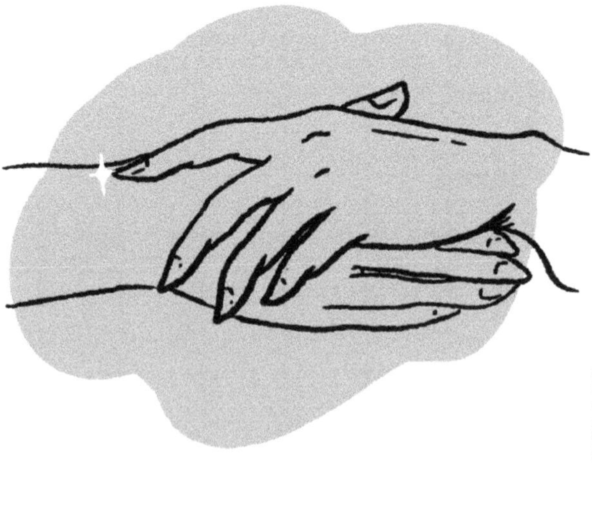

CHAPTER 8

Keep Calm & Love Your Heart

The Hidden Heart of PeriMenopause. One minute you're fine, the next your heart is pounding, your chest feels tight, and sleep? Forget it. Welcome to another curveball from PeriMenopause. You're not imagining things. You're not being dramatic. Your heart is feeling everything, literally and emotionally.

As oestrogen and progesterone decline, they take their calming effect with them. The result? Increased anxiety, disrupted sleep, and a cardiovascular system that suddenly seems to have a flair for drama.

But once you understand what's happening, you can do something about it and that's where this chapter comes in.

Hormones and Your Heart: What's Really Going On?

Let's get clinical for a moment.

Oestrogen affects neurotransmitters (aka hormone messengers) like serotonin and dopamine, which regulate mood, sleep, and stress resilience. It also supports blood vessel flexibility and healthy circulation. So when it drops your nervous system can shift into overdrive, even without a clear trigger.

Common symptoms include:

- Heart palpitations: Sudden fluttering, racing, or thudding sensations.
- Night sweats & vivid dreams: Often linked to heart function in Traditional Chinese Medicine (TCM).
- Increased anxiety or panic: Especially before bed or upon waking.
- Rising blood pressure or cholesterol: As oestrogen levels fall, vessel walls may stiffen, and cholesterol balance can shift.

And here's something no one tells you: heartbreak, grief, and unresolved emotional stress can amplify these physical symptoms.

TCM Insight: The Heart and Shen

In Traditional Chinese Medicine, the Heart is more than a pump. It's the home of the Shen (your spirit, emotional clarity, and consciousness).

When the Heart becomes overwhelmed (from hormonal shifts, emotional overload, or disturbed sleep) the Shen can become restless. The result? Anxiety, palpitations, insomnia, weepiness, or feeling emotionally fragile.

TCM also links excessive facial sweating (especially with emotional stress) to a Heart-Lung imbalance.

Bonus Insight: The Lungs help regulate fluids and the surface of the skin. Grief or unresolved sadness can weaken Lung energy, leading to unexpected sweating or breathlessness.

What's beautiful about TCM is this: One symptom often reflects multiple layers - physical, emotional, and hormonal.

The Press-Pulsate-Pause Method™ for Heart Health

Advanced Acupressure to steady the pulse, calm the spirit, and soothe your nervous system (Refer to Chapter 3 for full instructions).

- **Heart 7 神门 (Shén Mén)**
    - Inner wrist crease, aligned with the pinky.
    - Nourishes the Heart, soothes emotional overwhelm and anxiety, and improves sleep. You won't be crying at E.V.E.R.Y single thing!

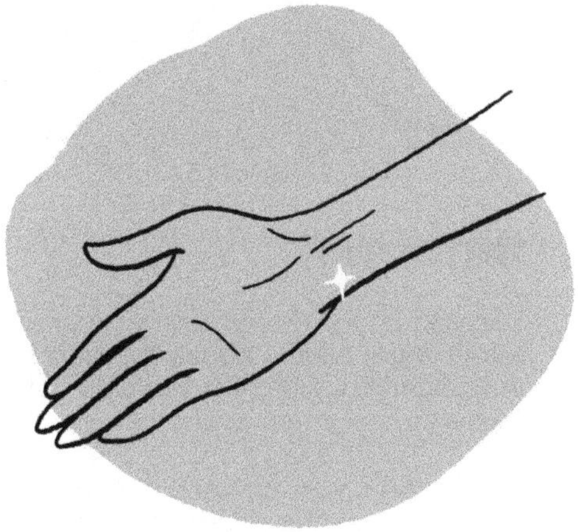

AcuWarrior™ Tip: Gently apply while breathing slowly.

- **Pericardium 6 内关 (Nèi Guān)**
    - Three finger-widths above the wrist crease, between the tendons.
    - Regulates heart rhythm, calms palpitations, eases nausea, and grounds your emotions. Start saying "NO" and protect your boundaries!

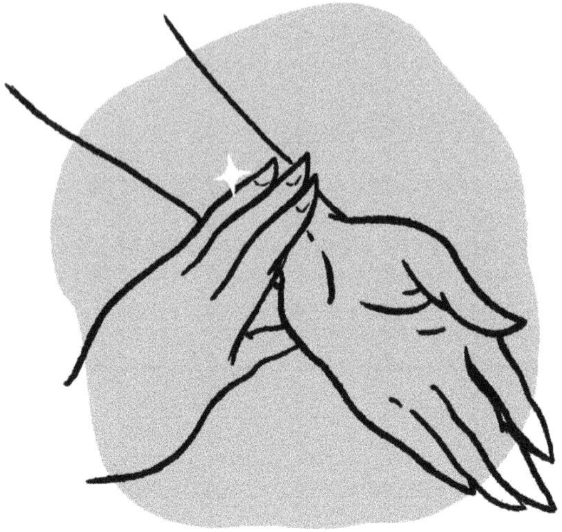

- **Lung 7 列缺 (Liè Quē)**
    - Located on the thumb side of your wrist, about one and a half finger widths above the wrist crease. You'll find it in a slight dip, just off to the side of the bone. It's often easier to feel when your palm is turned towards you.
    - Opens the chest, clears emotional grief, and helps manage sweating. Eases breathlessness, being teary, or sweating from stress.

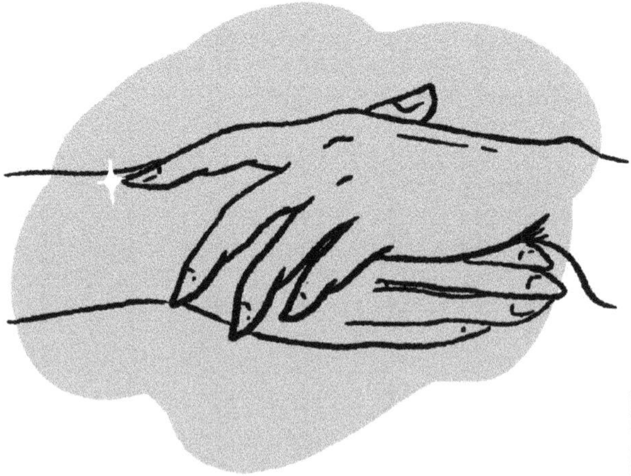

AcuWarrior™ Reminder: "Two minutes a day keeps the peri away."

AromaAcu Therapy™ for the Heart

(Refer to Chapter 3 for how to use oils safely)

These heart-loving oils work through your limbic brain - the emotional centre that responds to scent within seconds or a few hours.

- Rose - Sacred in both TCM and Persian culture. Emotionally uplifting, spiritually anchoring, and a classic tonic for the Heart.
- Lavender - Calms the nervous system and gently lowers blood pressure.
- Ylang Ylang - Reduces cortisol and softens emotional agitation.
- Petitgrain - Settles an overactive mind without making you drowsy.

Science says: Aromatherapy supports emotional regulation via the hypothalamus, influencing hormones and the stress response.

Supplement Support for Heart Health

Always consult a healthcare professional or book a consultation with me.

- Magnesium Glycinate: Calms the nervous system and supports heart rhythm.
- CoQ10: Vital for heart energy and blood pressure regulation, especially post-40.
- Omega-3 (EPA/DHA): Reduces inflammation and supports cholesterol balance.
- Hawthorn Berry: A traditional Heart tonic in both Chinese and Western herbalism.

Combined Healing Breath Ritual & Affirmation: Calm Heart, Calm Body

For when your pulse races or your chest feels tight.

Ritual Steps:

1. Place your left hand over your heart, right hand just beneath it.
2. Inhale through the nose for a count of 4.
3. Visualise golden light expanding from your heart with every exhale.
4. Whisper this affirmation to yourself: "My heart is steady. My breath is calm. I feel safe at this moment."
5. Repeat for 3-5 breath cycles. Stay until the body feels softer.

A grateful heart is a strong heart.

Quick Wins

- Walk in nature - it lowers blood pressure and regulates your nervous system.
- Sip rose or hawthorn tea for emotional steadiness. (Check medical suitability).
- Avoid caffeine if you experience racing heart symptoms.
- Journal to clear emotional heaviness from your chest.

Gratitude Prompt

Your heart isn't just pumping blood, it's holding your stories. This week, ask yourself when did my heart feel most at ease? What (or who) helped it feel safe, even for a moment?

Take a breath. Place your hand on your chest. Feel the rhythm that keeps showing up for you, even when life gets loud. Now whisper a thank you. Your heart hears it.

Persian Wisdom

"What the heart holds, the tongue will speak."

دل هر چه خواهد زبان گوید

Transliteration: Del har che khahad zaban guyad.

Meaning: When emotions remain unprocessed, they often leak out in unexpected ways. Regulate the heart, and your words (and your life) flow with more grace.

Let's Keep Talking: *You don't need to suffer in silence. Tag @AcuCareClinicUK and use* **#PocketPeri** - *I'd love to see how you support your heart.*

Next Up: *All things sleep hygiene & fatigue because a calm heart deserves deep rest.*

CHAPTER 9

Sleep & Fatigue

Reclaiming Rest When You're Running on Empty

You're not just tired. You're running on hormonal mayhem!

We've all been there: lying awake at 2am, mind racing, body restless, wondering if sleep is a distant memory from your former life. Congratulations! You've unlocked a new level of PeriMenopause where your hormones throw a surprise party at night, and you're not even invited to sleep through it.

The good news? It's not all in your head. And no, you're not just *"getting older."*

Hormonal changes during PeriMenopause genuinely disrupt your sleep architecture. But with the right support, you can get your sleep back on track.

Why PeriMenopause Wrecks Your Sleep (and Zaps Your Energy)

Hormones are your body's natural sleep conductors and, when they start misfiring, everything goes offbeat.

During PeriMenopause:

- Progesterone drops, making it harder to fall asleep or stay asleep.
- Oestrogen fluctuates, contributing to night sweats, anxiety, and hot flushes.
- Cortisol (your stress hormone) rises at the wrong time, making you alert when you should be winding down.
- Melatonin (your body's natural sleep hormone) dips, delaying your sleep-wake rhythm.

It's not surprising you feel like you've aged 10 years overnight.

You Might Be Experiencing:

- Waking at 1-3 a.m. and struggling to get back to sleep.
- Night sweats or hot flushes that leave your sheets drenched.
- Tired but wired: feeling exhausted all day, but suddenly alert at bedtime.
- Crashing mid-afternoon, only to get a second-wind at 9 p.m.
- Burnout that feels emotional, hormonal, and physical all at once.

Sound familiar? You're not alone and you're not falling apart. Your body is calling for balance, not punishment.

The TCM View: Why Sleep Disruption Runs Deeper Than You Think

In Traditional Chinese Medicine (TCM), sleep is governed by the Heart, Liver, and Kidneys, each with their own emotional and physical role. These organs don't just pump blood or filter waste. They're also responsible for:

- **Heart**: Housing the Shen (mind/spirit). If disrupted, you feel anxious or have disturbed sleep.

- **Liver**: Regulating blood and emotions. If Liver energy is stagnant or overheated, you wake between 1-3 a.m.

- **Kidneys**: Storing your life force. Weak Kidney energy leads to fatigue, restlessness, and poor recovery.

You may remember from Chapter 8 that the Heart governs not only circulation but also sleep quality. When the Heart is overheated or when emotional stress hasn't been processed then sleep disturbances often follow.

The Press-Pulsate-Pause Method™ for Sleep & Fatigue

(Refer to Chapter 3 for full instructions)

When your nervous system is overstimulated and your hormones are fluctuating, acupressure can help reset your rhythm. Use these points before bed or if you wake in the night:

- **Kidney 1 涌泉 (Yǒng Quán)**
    - Found on the sole of the foot, about one-third of the way down from the base of the toes towards the heel, in the soft dip between the ball of the foot and the arch, roughly in line with the second and third toes.
    - Grounds the nervous system, helps descend excess energy.

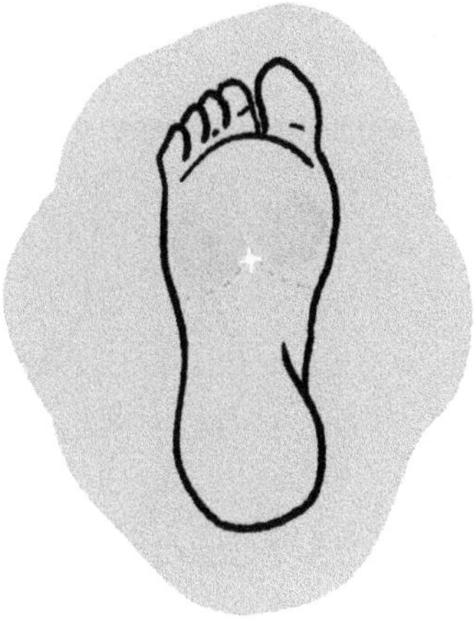

- **Heart 7 神门 (Shén Mén)**
    - On the wrist crease, in line with the pinky finger.
    - Calms the mind, eases anxiety and emotional restlessness.

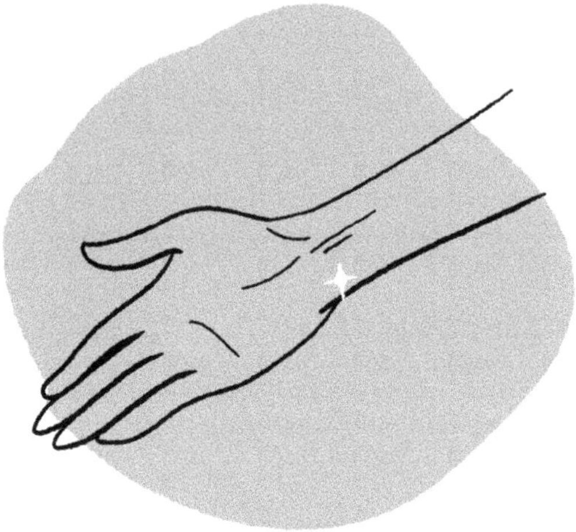

AcuWarrior™ Tip: Lavender essential oil is one of the very few oils safe enough to use in tiny amounts directly on skin. In this case, simply dab a drop of 100% pure lavender oil onto your fingertip and apply gently. If you have any medical conditions, always check with your practitioner first.

- **Liver 3 太冲 (Tài Chōng)**
    - On top of the foot, in the webbing between the big toe and second toe.
    - Balances emotional excess, supports deep sleep between 1-3 a.m.

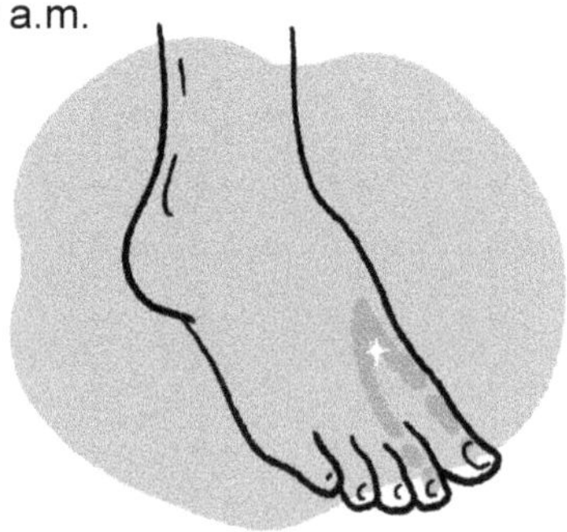

AcuWarrior™ Reminder:

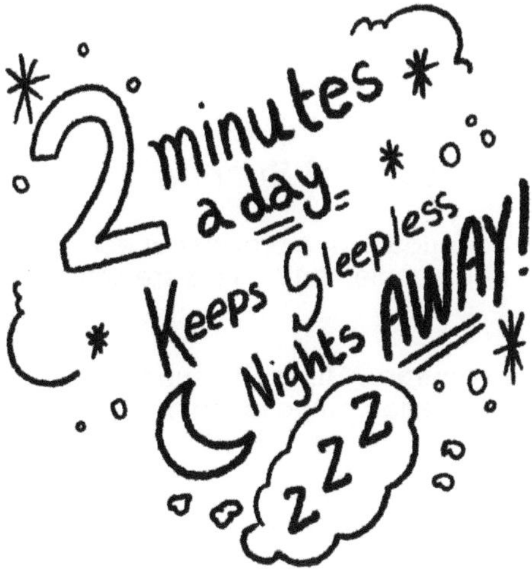

AromaAcu Therapy™ for Deep Rest

(Refer to Chapter 3 for how to use oils safely)

My AromaAcu Therapy™ combines calming essential oils with the previously mentioned acupressure points, perfect for winding down before bed.

Recommended oils:

- Lavender - Sedative, heart-soothing.
- Roman Chamomile - Eases restlessness and tension.
- Frankincense - Grounds scattered thoughts.
- Rose - Emotional comfort for sleep disturbed by stress or sadness.

Safety Note:

Always keep essential oils away from children and pets (especially cats and dogs) and avoid placing oils directly on fur or bedding. While I truly believe applying diluted, prescription oil blends to the skin can be helpful in the right context, I don't recommend self-prescribing. As explained in

Chapter 3, essential oil safety is complex and what works for one person won't suit another. If you'd like personalised guidance, seek a qualified aromatherapist, or you're welcome to book an online consultation with me. I support patients worldwide.

Supplements & Nutritional Support

Always check with your healthcare provider or book a consultation with me before starting new supplements. Here are commonly supported options:

Magnesium (The Relaxation Mineral) - supports sleep, nervous system health, and muscle relaxation. Choose the right form:

Type	Best for	Notes
Magnesium Glycinate	Sleep & anxiety	No laxative effect; gentle on stomach
Magnesium Citrate	Sleep + constipation	Mild laxative; good for sluggish digestion
Magnesium Threonate	Brain fog & cognition	Crosses blood-brain barrier
Magnesium Malate	Fatigue & muscle tension	Energising yet relaxing

Stick to recommended doses, more isn't always better.

Healing Breath Ritual for Liver & Sleep Regulation

Ritual steps:

1. Place your right hand on your right lower ribs (liver), left hand on your chest.
2. Inhale slowly into your chest, then down to your right hand.
3. Exhale with a gentle sigh, imagining heat and frustration leaving the body.
4. Whisper: "Thank you for helping me rest and renew."

Quick Wins

- Cool your bedroom: 16-18°C is the sweet spot.
- No screens 30 minutes before bed: blue light delays melatonin.
- Read or stretch instead of scrolling.
- No caffeine after 2 p.m. (yes, even the sneaky green tea).
- Use scent strategically: lavender mist, cotton-wool oil near pillow.
- Track your patterns: journal wake-up times, triggers, or helpful habits.

Affirmation

"I give myself permission to rest, recharge, and receive the sleep I deserve."

Gratitude Prompt

Before you collapse into bed tonight, pause and ask what's one thing I did today that supported my rest, no matter how small? When did I feel even a flicker of ease, comfort, or quiet in my body?

Write it down. Whisper "thank you". You're not lazy, you're healing. This is how we rebuild rest, one gentle moment at a time.

Persian Wisdom

"Sleep is not a weakness . It is the strength behind all strength."

خواب ضعف نیست، قدرتی‌ست که پشت همهٔ قدرت‌هاست

Transliteration: Khaab za'f nist, ghovvati-st ke posht-e hameye ghovvat-ha-st

Meaning: Sleep is sacred. Don't dismiss it. Rest is how your body recovers, your mind heals, and your spirit strengthens.

***Let's Keep Talking**: Tag me using **#PocketPeri** and mention @AcuCareClinicUK. I'd love to see your rest rituals and bedtime wins. QR code to socials*

@ACUCARE_CLINIC_UK

***Next Up**: It's all about beating the heat of PeriMenopause. Let's get you cool, grounded, and confident again.*

CHAPTER 10

Cool, Calm, and Collected

Beating the Heat of PeriMenopause

Welcome to the Unexpected Sauna!

Suddenly sweating through your clothes? Waking up drenched for no good reason? Feeling like someone turned the internal thermostat up to 100? You're not melting. You're PeriMenopausal.

Hot flushes and night sweats are among the most visible symptoms of hormonal shifts, but they're not just about temperature. They're tied to your nervous system, stress levels, emotional heat, and sometimes even grief. And while it might feel like your body's working against you, there's a way to stay cool, inside and out.

Why the Heat Hits So Hard

Blame your beautiful brain. Specifically, your hypothalamus, the part of your brain that controls your body's thermostat.

During PeriMenopause:

- Oestrogen declines, confusing your hypothalamus and triggering false heat alarms.
- Cortisol surges (hello, stress), which fans the flames even more.
- Blood vessels dilate, causing that sudden, overwhelming flush.
- Night sweats disrupt sleep, which creates a cycle of fatigue and more flushes (as we saw in Chapter 9).

It's not just uncomfortable. It's exhausting. Trust me, I know this one all too well.

The TCM Take: When Heat Rises, Calm Must Follow

In Traditional Chinese Medicine (TCM), hot flushes are often the result of:

- **Heart Fire**: Emotional heat and overstimulation of the Heart.
- **Liver Heat or Stagnation**: Frustration, stress, and repressed emotions creating internal agitation.
- **Kidney Yin Deficiency**: Not enough cooling, nourishing fluids to balance rising heat.

You may recall from Chapter 8 that the Heart governs circulation and sweat, while the Liver processes emotion. When both are out of balance, the body overheats and the result is a PeriMenopausal rollercoaster of steam, sweat, and short tempers.

But the solution isn't suppression, it's regulation.

The Press-Pulsate-Pause Method™ for Cooling Relief

(Refer to Chapter 3 for full instructions)

Use these points daily or during a hot flush to help regulate your body's internal thermostat.

- **Kidney 1 涌泉 (Yǒng Quán)**
  - On the sole of the foot, just below the ball.
  - Grounds heat and brings down excess energy/heat.

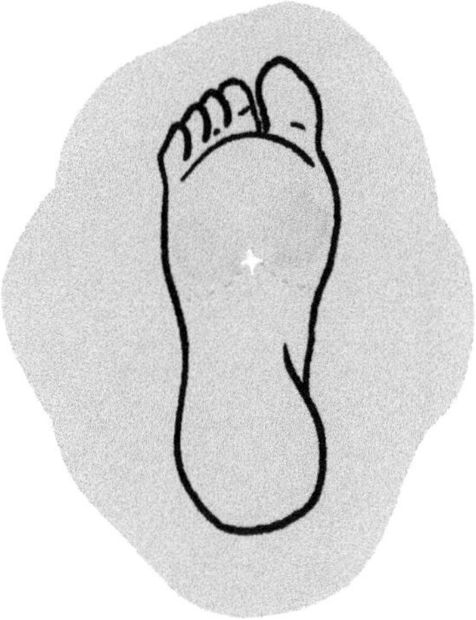

- **Pericardium 6 内关 (Nèi Guān)**
  - Three finger-widths above the wrist crease, between the tendons.
  - Calms emotional heat, eases palpitations, and cools the chest.

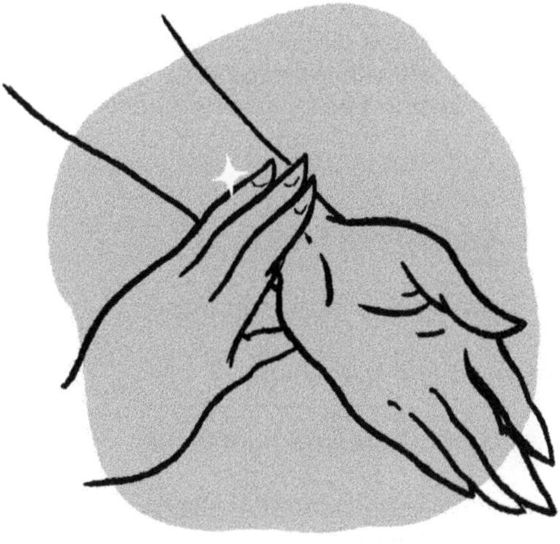

- **Large Intestine 4 合谷 (Hé Gǔ)**
    - Between thumb and index finger.
    - Moves stagnation and clears heat.
    - Avoid if pregnant.

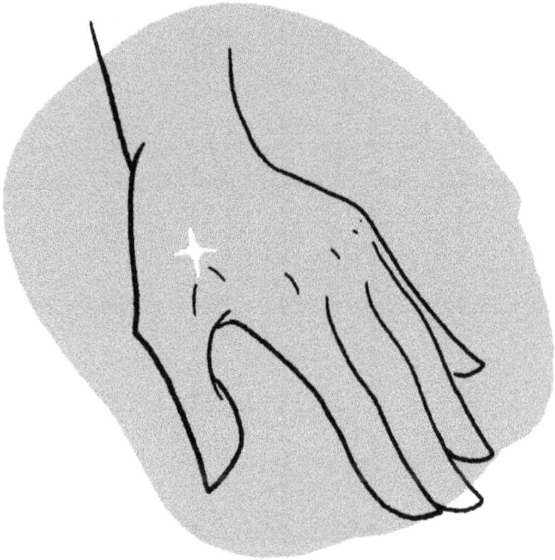

AromaAcu Therapy™ for Cooling the Flame

(Refer to Chapter 3 for how to use oils safely)

Essential oils are powerful allies when your body feels like it's boiling from the inside. When paired with acupressure, they can help calm the mind, cool the skin, and support emotional regulation.

Recommended oils:

- Peppermint - Cooling and refreshing.
- Lavender - Calming and heat-clearing.
- Rose - Luxurious and hydrating.
- Clary Sage - Gently hormone-supportive.

Safety Note: Please don't apply essential oils directly to your skin unless under the guidance of a qualified aromatherapist. While I do use diluted, prescription blends for my clients in-clinic, I don't recommend self-prescribing. If you'd like support, you're welcome to book a virtual consultation with me. I support patients worldwide.

BONUS DIY Cooling Mist (For Daytime Use)

When the flush hits during the day, a gentle mist can feel like magic.

Cooling Mist Recipe:

- 100 ml distilled water.
- 3 drops peppermint essential oil.
- 3 drops lavender essential oil.
- Optional: 1 drop rose or clary sage oil.

Mix in a spray bottle, shake well before each use, and spritz lightly on your face and neck. Avoid direct contact with the eyes.

Safety Note: Patch test before use. Always spray into the air and walk through it (Just like that episode of Friends. If you know, you know who and what I'm talking about. Wink, wink.)

The Layering Rule (Your New Anti-Flush Philosophy)

Hot one minute, freezing the next? Welcome to the PeriMenopause paradox.

Here's the TCM-informed rule: Never remove layers while you're sweating.

Why? Because your pores are open, and exposure to cold or wind can lead to what TCM calls a "wind invasion", weakening your immune system and leading to chills, aches, or low energy.

Do:

- Remove layers before sweating starts.
- Keep lightweight layers handy (cotton, bamboo).
- Avoid cold drafts or direct fans on your neck.

"Fans are for cooling the room. Not blowing your immune system out of balance."

AcuWarrior™ Tip: When the heat hits, take charge like the queen you are. Preparation is power. Arm yourself with cooling rituals so you can move through your day (and night) with grace, not gritted teeth.

Healing Breath Ritual for A Cooling Wave

Use this anytime you feel overheated, physically or emotionally.

Ritual steps:

1. Sit comfortably with one hand on your heart and the other on your lower abdomen.
2. Inhale slowly, imagining cool air washing through your chest and belly.
3. As you exhale, picture steam rising and dissipating.
4. Whisper: "I am calm, collected, balanced, and refreshed."
5. Repeat for 2-3 rounds, or as long as it takes to feel re-centred.

Quick Wins

- Drink chrysanthemum tea - A TCM favourite for reducing internal heat.
- Eat hydrating foods - Watermelon, cucumber, celery.
- Sip cool (not cold) water - Gulping ice water can cause more imbalance.
- Moisture-wicking sleepwear - Choose breathable bamboo or cotton.
- Keep a bowl of room-temp water nearby, dip a cloth in, apply, then dry off gently.
- Blot, don't rub - Use cooled cloth or blotting papers on the face.
- Try flaxseed or tofu - Add ground flaxseed to smoothies or breakfast bowls, or use tofu in stir-fries and soups. Both contain gentle phytoestrogens to help balance oestrogen levels over time.

Affirmation

"I navigate my body's rhythms with grace and confidence. I am in control, calm, and empowered."

Gratitude Prompt

After reading this chapter, take a moment to honour your body's signals, even the sweaty, inconvenient, ones. Ask yourself what's one moment I stayed calm under heat - literal or emotional? What helped me feel more at ease this week?

This isn't just about cooling down. It's about turning toward your body with compassion, even when it's turning up the heat.

Write it down. Let that be enough for today.

Persian Wisdom

"Heat may rise, but grace keeps us grounded. Emotional control and balance is the key to calm."

حرارت بالا می‌رود، اما وقار ما را در زمین نگه می‌دارد

Transliteration: Haraarat baalaa miravad, ammaa veghaar maa raa dar zamin negah midaarad

Meaning: Let your power rise, not your panic. True calm comes from within.

Let's Keep Talking: *Tag me using* ***#PocketPeri*** *and mention @AcuCareClinicUK. I'd love to see your cooling rituals and calming wins.*

Next Up: *Your body's been overheating and now it's undercharging! Next, we explore why PeriMenopause fatigue hits so hard, and how to build your energy back (without caffeine or chaos).*

CHAPTER 11

From Fatigue to Fierce

Your PeriMenopause Energy Reboot

You're NOT lazy. One minute you're powering through your to-do list. The next? You're flat on the sofa wondering if blinking counts as cardio.

Fatigue in PeriMenopause isn't your average tired. It's deep, unpredictable, and sometimes relentless. You might be doing "all the right things", sleeping, eating, even exercising but your body still feels like it's running on 5% battery. And the worst part? Most people don't understand just how draining this phase can be.

This chapter isn't about hustle culture or pushing through. It's about understanding the real reasons behind your exhaustion and offering science-backed, holistic, ways to feel like yourself again, just fiercer.

Western Insight: Why Am I So Tired?

Let's get straight to it: PeriMenopause fatigue is not your fault. It's the result of a complex hormonal shuffle and other factors that affect your body's ability to sustain energy.

Common Culprits Include:

- **Hormonal Shifts** - Fluctuating oestrogen and progesterone disrupt sleep and energy balance. Cortisol (your stress hormone) may surge in response, leading to wired-but-tired burnout.

- **Thyroid Function** - Your thyroid slows down during PeriMenopause for some women, triggering fatigue, brain fog, and cold sensitivity.

- **Anaemia** - Heavy periods during this phase often lead to iron deficiency. Classic signs: exhaustion, dizziness, and breathlessness.

- **Blood Sugar Swing** - Hormonal changes affect insulin sensitivity, meaning sugar highs (and crashing lows) happen more easily.

Know Your Numbers: When to Test

You don't need to guess what's happening under the surface. Ask your doctor about checking these levels, or some practitioners (like myself) offer home test kits via consultation if you prefer a personalised approach.

Recommended tests:

- Thyroid Panel - TSH, T4 (and ideally T3 + thyroid antibodies).

- Iron & Ferritin - Ask specifically for ferritin, it's often missed.

- Vitamin D & B12 - Both are essential for energy production.

- Blood Sugar Levels - Glucose or HbA1c to rule out insulin resistance.

TCM Insight: The Three Vital Systems

In Traditional Chinese Medicine, fatigue often stems from weakened function in three core systems. Let's translate that into modern terms:

- **Liver System**: Linked to blood flow, detoxification, and emotional processing. When overloaded? You feel sluggish and irritable. Eat bitter greens like rocket and dandelion; prioritise hydration.
- **Spleen System**: Regulates digestion and nutrient absorption which is crucial for steady energy. Stick to warm, cooked foods. Avoid raw, cold meals that stress your gut.
- **Kidney System**: Associated with long-term vitality and hormonal resilience.

Black beans, walnuts, sesame seeds and naps. Yes, naps count as medicine.

The Press-Pulsate-Pause Method™ for Energy Reboot

(Refer back to Chapter 3 for full instructions)

You can use one point at a time, all at once, one side or both, whatever feels right but remember: less is more.

- **Stomach 36 足三里 (Zú Sān Lǐ)-** *One of my favourite points!*
    - Four finger-widths below your kneecap, one finger-width from the outer edge of your shinbone.
    - Supports digestion, improves circulation, and restores your energy reserves.

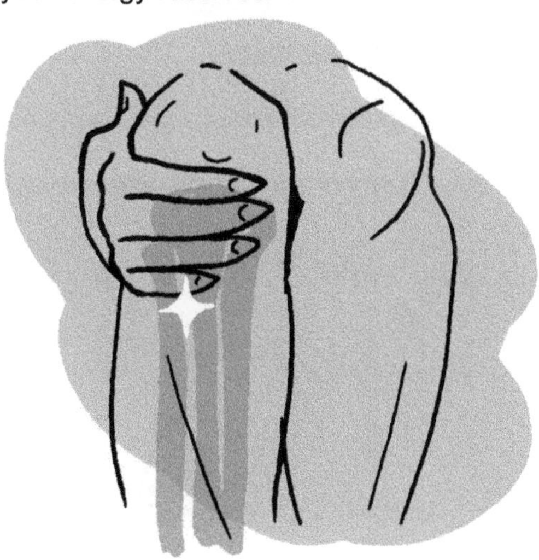

Legend has it that regular stimulation of this point gives you the strength to walk three miles without breaking a sweat. Let me know if it works for you. I'd love to hear your three-mile story!

- **Kidney 1 涌泉 (Yǒng Quán)**
    - Found on the sole of the foot, about one-third of the way down from the base of the toes towards the heel, in the soft dip between the ball of the foot and the arch, roughly in line with the second and third toes.
    - Recharges depleted energy and grounds nervous tension.

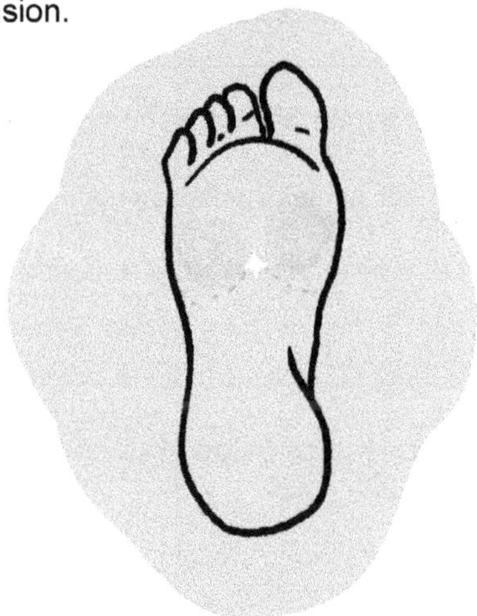

- **Pericardium 6 内关 (Nèi Guān)**
    - Three finger-widths above the inner wrist crease.
    - Relieves stress and boosts heart-energy connection.

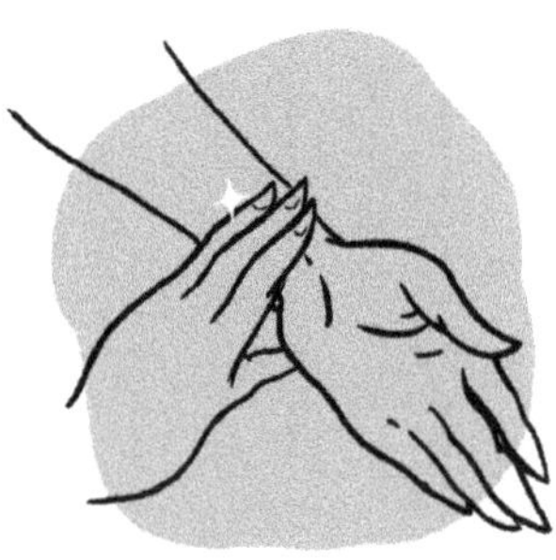

- **Large Intestine 4 合谷 (Hé Gǔ)**
    - In the web between thumb and index finger.
    - Revs up circulation and relieves head heaviness.
    - Avoid during pregnancy.

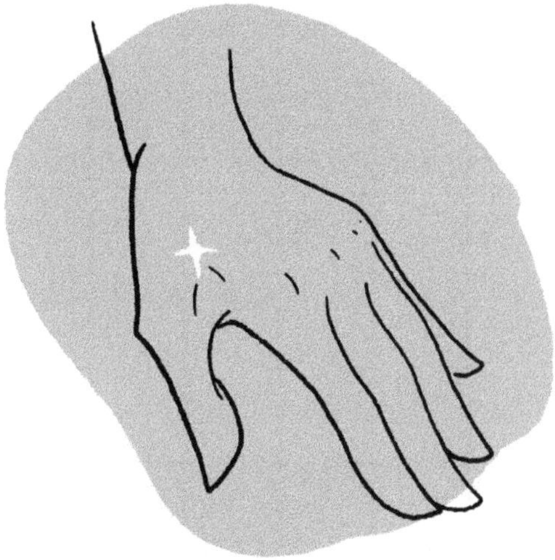

- **Liver 3 太冲 (Tài Chōng)**
    - Between the big toe and second toe.
    - Eases irritability and clears hormonal stagnation (i.e. poor blood flow).

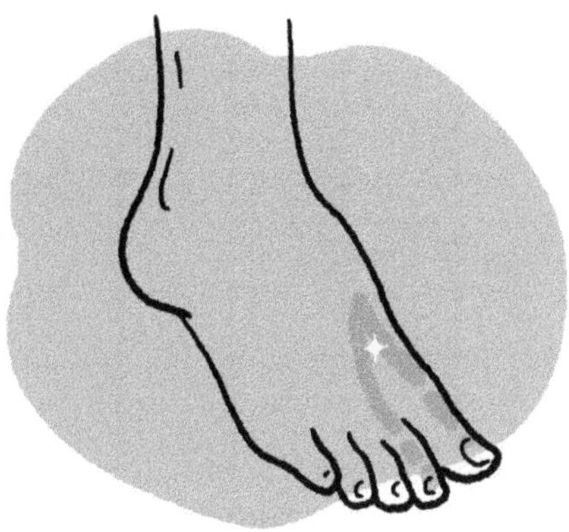

AromaAcu Therapy™ for Energy Support

(Refer to Chapter 3 for how to use oils safely)

Recommended oils:

- Peppermint - Sharpens focus and clears mental fog.
- Rosemary - Improves blood flow and supports brain clarity.
- Lemon - Brightens mood and fights fatigue with a zesty uplift.
- Healing Breath Ritual to Recharge and Renew

Ritual steps:

1. Sit comfortably with one hand on your chest, the other on your lower abdomen.
2. Inhale slowly, feeling your belly rise.
3. Exhale even slower, releasing tension and visualising your energy returning.
4. Say silently or aloud: "I breathe in strength and vitality. I exhale exhaustion and stress."

AcuWarrior™ Reminder: "Two minutes a day keeps the peri away."

Quick Wins

- Eat smart - Protein: Eggs, tofu, lentils. Healthy fats: Avocados, nuts. Slow carbs: Quinoa, sweet potato. Adaptogens: Nettle or ginseng tea but check for medication interactions.
- Move gently - 10 mins of stretching, yoga, or even squats while brushing your teeth. Find something joyful like dancing, boxing, or a slow walk with music

- Box Breathing - Inhale for 4. Hold for 4. Exhale for 4. Hold for 4. Repeat for 2-3 mins to reset your nervous system.

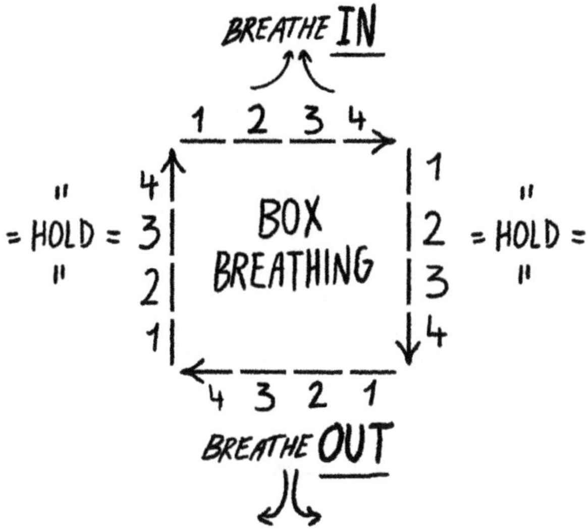

- Consider supplements - Iron (if testing low). Magnesium. Vitamin D & B12. (Always check with your practitioner or your GP before starting new supplements).

Affirmation

"I honour my body's rhythm. I nourish my energy with compassion and embrace each day with strength."

Gratitude Prompt

You made it to the end of this chapter so that's already a win! Ask yourself what's one thing I did this week that supported my energy, even in a small way? Where can I offer myself more compassion instead of criticism?

This isn't about doing more. It's about recognising the quiet victories such as listening to your body and honouring its pace. Write it down. Then rest. Fiercely.

Persian Wisdom

"The body is a garden, and rest is its water. Tend it with care, and it will bloom."

بدن باغی است، و استراحت آبیاری آن است. با دلسوزی آن را پرورش بده

Transliteration: Badan bâghi ast, va esteraahat aabiyaari-e ân ast. Bâ delsozzi ân râ parvaresh bedeh

Meaning: Your energy is renewable but only if you protect it. Rest is not laziness, it's life-giving.

AcuWarrior™ Tip: Energy isn't just physical, it's emotional, too. Music can shift your entire state in seconds. Whether it's a power anthem or a calming instrumental, keep a playlist that matches your mood or lifts it (We've got something special coming in Chapter 17 so stay tuned).

***Let's Keep Talking**: Tag me using **#PocketPeri** and mention @AcuCareClinicUK. I'd love to know how this chapter has helped you.*

***Next Up**: Get ready to meet your gut and your hormones' least predictable best friend. Gut Health & PeriMenopause - A Love-Hate Relationship.*

CHAPTER 12

Gut Instincts

Mastering Digestive Health When Your Stomach Won't Stay Quiet

Let's be honest, no one talks enough about the bloating, burping, or bathroom dramas of PeriMenopause. But if your gut has gone from calm to chaotic, you're not imagining it. Your hormones and your digestion are in constant conversation and sometimes, they're arguing loudly.

During PeriMenopause, it's not just your mood swings that surprise you. There's also the gurgling stomach, sudden food sensitivities, and that suspicious tightness in your waistband after half a salad. This chapter helps you reclaim control from the inside out, with science-backed insights and Traditional Chinese Medicine (TCM) wisdom that doesn't involve giving up all your favourite foods.

Western Insight: The Gut-Hormone Connection

Your gut isn't just a digestion station. It's an entire ecosystem. This microbiome, made up of trillions of bacteria, enzymes, and immune cells, influences everything from mood to metabolism. And yes, it plays a major role in how your body handles hormones like oestrogen.

Oestrogen is metabolised through the liver and excreted via the gut. When your digestion slows or your microbiome is out of balance (a common issue in PeriMenopause), oestrogen can recirculate in the body rather than being cleared out efficiently. This can contribute to symptoms like bloating, mood swings, weight gain, and even skin flare-ups.

Did You Know? Some bacteria in your gut produce enzymes (especially one group called the estrobolome) that help break down oestrogen. An unhealthy gut microbiome can reduce these enzymes, contributing to hormonal chaos.

Know Your Numbers: Tests That Can Help

If your gut symptoms feel persistent or severe, it's worth investigating. Here are a few things you might want to ask your doctor about - or discuss with a practitioner (like myself) who offers easy home testing kits via consultation:

- **Comprehensive Stool Test** - To assess gut bacteria, inflammation, parasites, or yeast overgrowth.
- **SIBO Test** - Breath test to check for small intestinal bacterial overgrowth, which can cause bloating and gas.
- **Food Sensitivity Testing** - Can identify if certain foods are creating low-grade inflammation or discomfort.
- **Oestrogen Metabolites** - To check how efficiently your gut and liver are processing hormones.

You don't need to test everything at once, but knowing what's happening inside gives you the power to act with precision.

TCM Insight: Dampness, Stress & the Digestive Duo

In Traditional Chinese Medicine, your Stomach and Spleen are responsible for digesting food, absorbing nutrients, and turning it all into usable energy (aka blood and vitality, the stuff that keeps you going).

When these organs are strong, you feel energised, clear-headed, and light.

When they're not? You feel heavy, foggy, bloated, and drained.

One key concept here is Dampness - a term that describes the accumulation of fluids and undigested food in the body. It's not about being "wet," but rather the kind of internal clogging that causes bloating, puffiness, loose stools, or stubborn belly fat.

Dampness is made worse by:

- Eating cold, raw foods (like smoothies, salads, iced drinks).
- Overthinking and worry (which TCM says weakens the Spleen).
- Late-night snacking or overeating.

TCM offers an antidote: Eat warm, easy-to-digest meals. Support the digestive fire. Protect your Spleen. Calm the mind.

The Press-Pulsate-Pause Method™ for Digestion

Advanced Acupressure to calm your gut and clear the bloat. You can use one point at a time, all at once, one side or both. Whatever feels right but remember: less is more.

(See Chapter 3 for full instructions.)

- **Stomach 36 足三里 (Zú Sān Lǐ)**
    - Location: Four finger-widths below your kneecap, one finger-width from the outer edge of your shinbone.
    - Supports digestion, reduces bloating, and boosts overall energy.

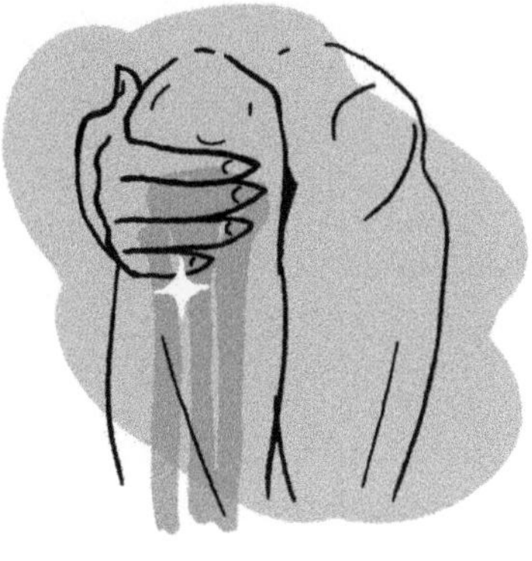

- **Conception Vessel 6 (Ren 6) 气海 (Qì Hǎi)-** *Another favourite point of mine!*

    - Two finger-widths below your belly button, in the centre line.

    - Strengthens digestive function and nourishes the gut.

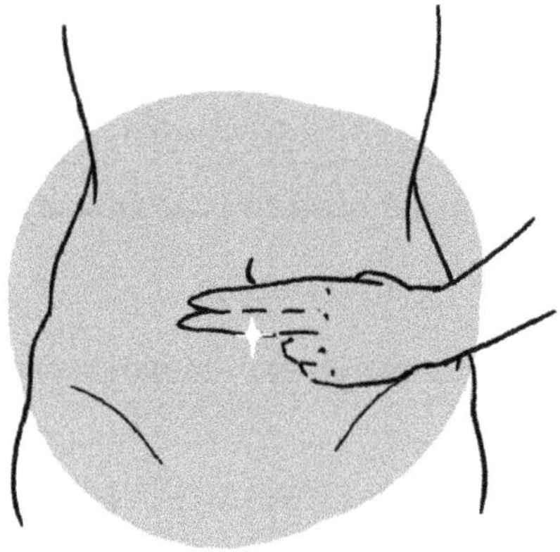

- **Spleen 9 阴陵泉 (Yīn Líng Quán)**

    - On the inner side of the lower leg, just below the knee crease, in a soft hollow.

    - Clears Dampness i.e. reduces water retention, and eases heaviness.

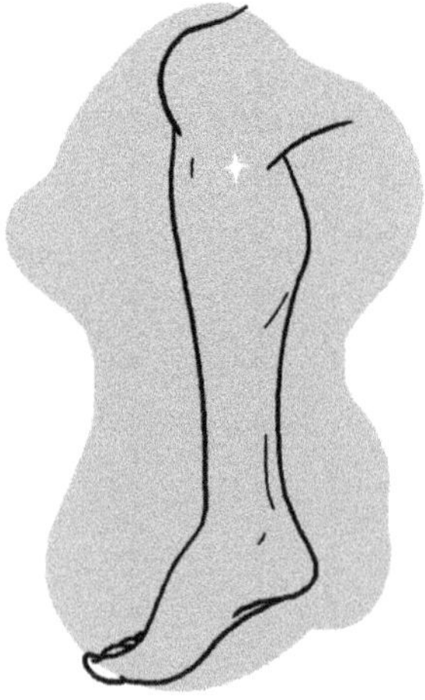

AromaAcu Therapy™ for Aiding Digestion

(Refer to Chapter 3 for how to use oils safely)

Essential oils can work beautifully alongside Advanced Acupressure. Their aromatic compounds activate the brain's limbic system helping to ease bloating, reduce nausea, and calm a stressed gut.

Recommended oils:

- Peppermint - Soothes cramps, gas, and bloating.
- Ginger - Warms the belly and aids sluggish digestion.
- Fennel - Relieves discomfort and supports motility.
- Chamomile - Calms gut tension and emotional stress.
- Cinnamon - A warming digestive and blood sugar balancer.

You may gently inhale during your acupressure practice - or place it near your setup for passive diffusion. Or simply place the infused damp cotton wool in a ceramic dish or on your desk while applying the Press-Pulsate-Pause Method™.

Bonus Tip:

Sip on a warm cup of ginger tea (or Sahar's Chai™) during your self-care ritual to support your gut from the inside out. Just maybe not right before bed. Your belly loves a brew, but your sleep might not!

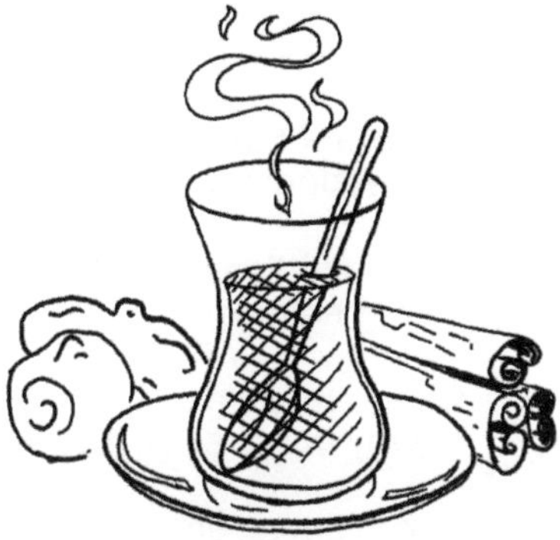

Healing Breath Ritual for Gut Instinct Reset

Ritual steps:

1. Place your hands over your lower abdomen.
2. Inhale through the nose, letting the breath expand your belly like a balloon.
3. Visualise warmth spreading from the stomach area to the sides

of your torso.

4. Exhale slowly and say: "Thank you for nourishing and energising my body."

Use this ritual before or after meals to calm the stomach and support smoother digestion.

Quick Wins

- Eat warm meals. Swap raw salads for soups, stews, and lightly steamed vegetables.
- Box Breathing: Inhale for 4, hold for 4, exhale for 4, hold for 4. Repeat for at least 3 sets. Great before meals.
- Try probiotics - such as Lactobacillus and Bifidobacterium strains. Look for multi-strain formulas or fermented foods like kefir, kimchi, and sauerkraut.
- Spices like ginger, cinnamon, turmeric can help warm the gut and reduce inflammation. (Hello! Sahar's Chai™!)
- Chew slowly. Mindful eating improves digestion instantly.
- Check for food sensitivities. Sometimes it's not what you eat, but how your gut reacts.
- Consider digestive bitters or enzymes. Speak to a practitioner before starting.
- Check supplement interactions. For example, ginseng may help energy but check if it suits your current meds.
- Watch the alcohol. Alcohol can disrupt the delicate balance of gut bacteria, increase intestinal permeability (a.k.a. "leaky gut"), and put extra stress on your liver which is already working hard to process hormonal changes during PeriMenopause.Try going alcohol-free for a week or two and see if you notice the difference.

Affirmation

"I listen to my gut. She's smarter than she gets credit for."

Gratitude Prompt

Your gut speaks and you need to listen. Ask yourself what's one thing I did this week that felt kind to my digestion? What food, habit, or moment of calm truly nourished me?

PeriMenopause isn't asking you to eat perfectly. It's inviting you to tune in, not tighten up. Write it down and thank your belly for trying to keep the peace.

Persian Wisdom

"The stomach is the house of all pain anc شکم، خانه‌ی همه دردها و همه آرامش‌هاست

تساهشمارآ همه و اهدرد همه ىهناخ ،مکش

Transliteration: Shekam, khaneye hame dardhā va hame ārameshhāst

Meaning: A healthy gut brings peace to the whole body but when upset, it speaks louder than any organ. Treat it with care.

Let's Keep Talking*: Tag me using* **#PocketPeri** *and mention @AcuCareClinicUK. I'd love to know your gut feeling about this chapter!*

Next Up*: We're talking immunity. From repeat infections to slow healing, PeriMenopause can challenge your body's defences. Let's explore how to stay resilient, inside and out.*

CHAPTER 13

The Immunity Advantage

Staying Resilient Through PeriMenopause

Ever noticed how the moment you finally stop for a break (say over the holidays) you get sick? That telltale sore throat, a bit of a sniffle, and before you know it, you're horizontal while everyone else is clinking mulled wine.

Now imagine this instead: you're the only one in the house who doesn't get the flu. And if you do catch it, you bounce back faster. That's the power of a well-tuned immune system, especially during PeriMenopause.

Hormones don't just affect your mood and your cycle. They impact how your body defends itself. So if you've been catching every bug going lately, it might not just be bad luck. Let's give your immune system the love it needs to keep you resilient and not just reactive.

Western Insight: Immunity in PeriMenopause

Your immune system is a complex, dynamic network and it loves balance. PeriMenopause brings natural hormonal shifts that can throw that balance off:

- **Oestrogen's Protective Role** - Oestrogen isn't just for reproduction - it plays a direct role in modulating immune function. As levels decline, your body becomes more vulnerable to inflammation, slower to recover, and more susceptible to infection. (Wondering why all of the sudden you've developed allergies and hay fever symptoms for the first time?!)

- **Stress and Cortisol Overload** - Chronic stress (hello, midlife chaos) increases cortisol, which can suppress immune activity and mess with inflammation control.

- **Gut Health and Immunity** - Around 70-80% of your immune cells live in your gut. That means what you digest influences what you fight. A disrupted microbiome (which is common in PeriMenopause) = reduced immunity.

Know Your Numbers: What to Test and Why

If you've been feeling run down or picking up every bug going ask your healthcare provider, or book a consultation with me, to explore the following tests:

- **Vitamin D** - Low levels are associated with higher risk of infection and fatigue.

- **Zinc** - Essential for immune cell communication and wound healing.

- **White blood cell count** - Reveals how active your immune system is.

- **CRP (C-Reactive Protein)** - Measures inflammation in the body.

Some practitioners (myself included) offer easy home test kits via consultation, making it simple to check your levels and rebalance accordingly.

TCM Insight - The Immunity Triangle

In Traditional Chinese Medicine (TCM), your immune strength is linked to three key organ systems:

- **Lungs** - Your first line of defence, linked to respiratory immunity and skin health.

- **Spleen** - Governs digestion and energy, both crucial to immunity.

- **Kidneys** - The root of vitality; when strong, your resilience improves.

TCM Note: The lungs "open into the skin," which is why dry or sensitive skin can be a reflection of weak immunity. We'll explore this more in our skin chapter later on.

The Press-Pulsate-Pause Method™ for Immunity

(Refer to Chapter 3 for full instructions)

Use these three Advanced Acupressure points to support your immune system gently and consistently. Remember: Prevention is better than cure, so feel free to practice these points daily. You can use one point at a time, all at once, one side or both, whatever feels right but remember: less is more in general.

- **Lung 7 列缺 (Liè Quē)**

    - Located on the thumb side of your wrist, about one and a half finger widths above the wrist crease. You'll find it in a slight dip, just off to the side of the bone. It's often easier to feel when your palm is turned towards you.

    - For strengthening respiratory defences, easing sore throats, and preventing colds.

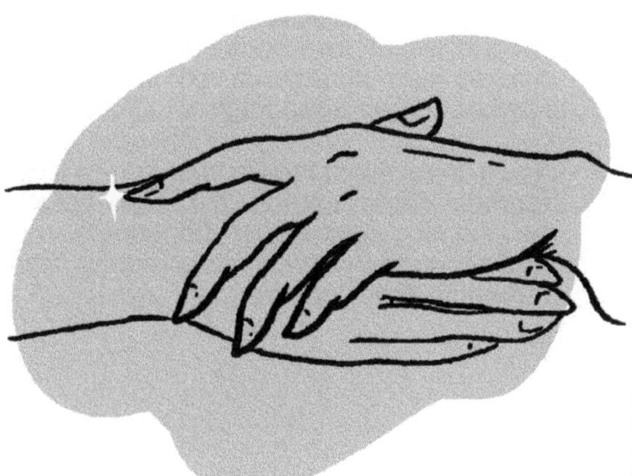

- **Stomach 36 足三里 (Zú Sān Lǐ)**
    - Four finger-widths below the kneecap, one finger-width to the outside of your shin bone.
    - Boosts energy, digestion, and resilience. Known as the "longevity point."

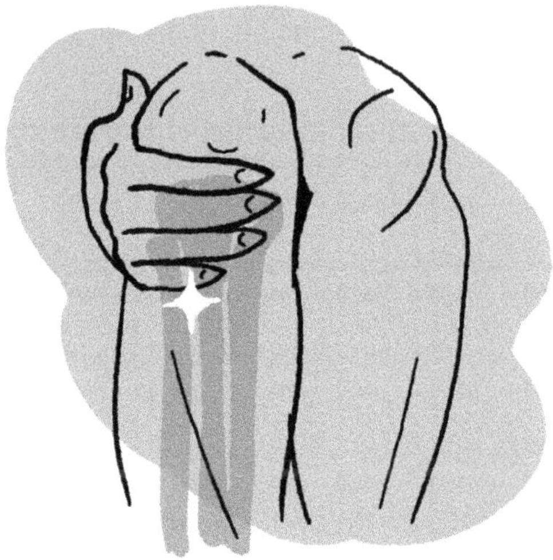

- **Kidney 27 俞府 (Shū Fǔ)**
    - Start by locating the centre of your chest, then feel for the soft dip just below your collarbone. Kidney 27 is roughly two finger-widths out from the centre, sitting in that dip near the edge of your breastbone, close to where your bra strap might sit, if you wear one).
    - You'll find a slight hollow there, that's Kidney 27! It's the topmost Kidney point on the chest, great for breathwork and calming tightness. It strengthens lungs and kidneys, and supports overall immune energy. This is your Immunity Activator point!

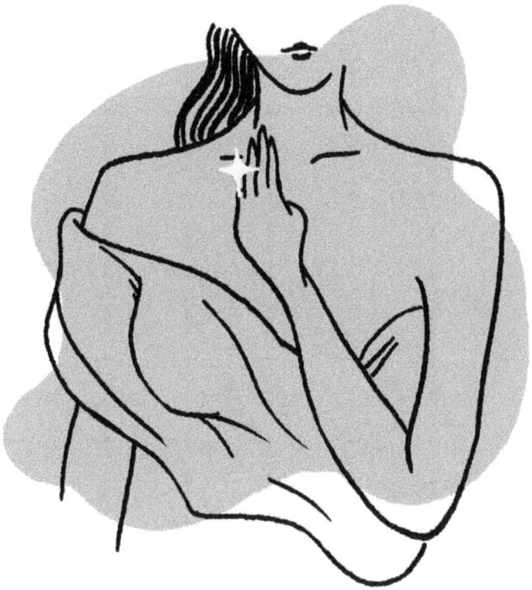

AromaAcu Therapy™ for Immunity

(Refer to Chapter 3 for how to use oils safely)

Combine the scent-power of essential oils with Advanced Acupressure for a deeper immune boost.

Recommended Oils:

- Eucalyptus - Opens airways and supports respiratory health.
- Tea Tree - Naturally antimicrobial.
- Lemon - Uplifts mood and helps cleanse the air.

Healing Breath Ritual for Immune Strength in Stillness

Ritual steps:

1. Sit or lay down comfortably with your hands on your chest.
2. As you inhale, imagine a protective glow forming around your body like a golden shield of resilience.

3. Exhale.

4. Affirm: "My body is strong, resilient, and ready to face the world."

Best Time: Morning or early evening, ideally when you feel calm. Prevention is better than cure.

AcuWarrior™ Reminder:

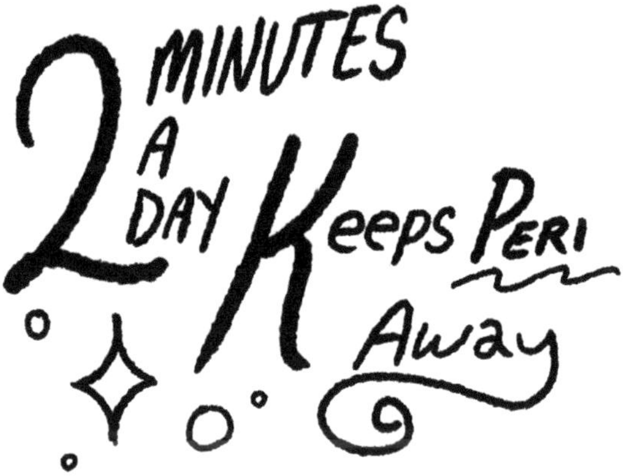

Quick Wins

- Eat the rainbow - Especially citrus fruits (Vitamin C), dark leafy greens, mushrooms, and fermented foods to nourish gut-immune connection.

- Sleep deeply - Your immune system repairs while you rest. Can't sleep? Check Chapter 9 for support.

- Use Advanced Acupressure - Press the points in the Press-Pulsate-Pause Method™ daily, even just for one minute each for gentle, natural immune support.

- Take probiotics - Helps balance gut bacteria - essential for a thriving immune system. Look for high-quality strains like Lactobacillus rhamnosus and Bifidobacterium lactis.

- Supplement smartly - Vitamin C (500-1000mg/day). Vitamin D3 (1000-2000 IU/day). Zinc (8mg/day). Check for interactions with any medications. If unsure, ask your healthcare provider or book a consultation with me.

- Sip smart - Enjoy a warm cup of lemon and ginger tea or Sahar's Chai™ during your evening wind-down. Your gut (and your mood) will thank you.

- Warm the core - If hot flushes allow, use a microwaveable wheat bag/hot water bottle over your lower abdomen (a method I recommend to many of my patients. It helps the body feel safe, relaxed, and resilient.) "A cold core invites colds. Keep your belly warm, your body happy."

- Avoid letting sweat dry on skin - Letting sweat dry (especially when outdoors) can weaken your defences. Change clothes or towel off when needed.

- Clean your phone - Your phone touches more bacteria than your toilet seat. Give it a wipe daily. PLEASE. Seriously, you wash your hands after work (I hope!), so why not clean your phone?

Affirmation

"My immune system is strong, vibrant, and protective. I nourish it with love and care."

Gratitude Prompt

Your body has your back even when you don't notice. Ask yourself what's one thing I did this week that supported my immune system, even in a small way? How can I thank my body for protecting me, even when I forget to protect it?

You're not fragile. You're fighting silent battles every day and still showing up. That deserves a pause, a breath, and a little praise.

Persian Wisdom

"Your health is like a house. Keep its windows clean, its foundation warm, and its doors strong against the winds."

تندرستی خانه‌ای است، با پنجره‌های تمیز، پایه‌های گرم، و درهایی استوار در برابر باد

Transliteration: Tandorosti khāneh-i ast, bā panjareh-hā-ye tamiz, pāyeh-hā-ye garm, va darhā-ye ostovār dar barābar-e bād.

Meaning: Your body, like a home, needs daily care (inside and out) to stay strong and open only to what serves you.

Myth-Busting - Immunity Edition

Myth #1: *"Hand sanitiser works better than washing your hands."*

The reality: Soap + water = top-tier bug-banisher.

Myth #2: *"You don't need to clean your phone unless you drop it."*

The reality: Think again. You carry it everywhere. Clean it daily - it's basically a germ-ridden pet.

Myth #3: *"If you eat enough greens, you don't need to supplement."*

Even nutrient-rich diets can miss key vitamins during hormone shifts.

***Let's Keep Talking**: Tag me using **#PocketPeri** and mention @AcuCareClinicUK. I'd love to hear how this chapter supported your inner strength and everyday resilience.*

***Next Up**: We're moving into the next layer of self-defence: muscle, bones, and joints. You'll learn how to protect your skeleton, ease joint pain, and embrace movement, even when your energy is on low battery mode.*

CHAPTER 14

Strong, Supple, and Steady

Your PeriMenopause Movement Manifesto

Forget everything you've ever heard about exercise being punishment for your body. During PeriMenopause, movement becomes your medicine. The daily ritual that supports your joints, strengthens your bones, balances your mood, and brings your energy back to life.

This isn't about sculpted abs or running marathons. It's about getting out of bed without pain, walking up stairs without breathlessness, and feeling strong enough to carry the shopping - or yourself - through the hormonal rollercoaster.

Movement can be gentle. It can be joyful. And yes, even two minutes a day can make a difference.

Western Insight: Why Movement Matters Now More Than Ever

Hormonal changes during PeriMenopause impact your muscles, joints, bones, metabolism, and mood:

- Loss of muscle mass begins in your 30s and accelerates with declining oestrogen. Less muscle = lower metabolism = more fatigue.

- Bone density decreases, especially in the spine, hips, and wrists. Oestrogen normally protects bones but, as it dips, bones become more fragile.

- Joint stiffness and pain become more common, often linked to inflammation, weight gain, and cortisol (your stress hormone) running the show.

- Mood and mental health also take a hit. Exercise boosts endorphins, regulates insulin, and helps reduce anxiety, depression, and brain fog.

Exercise isn't a fix, it's a foundation. Even small daily movements can recalibrate your nervous system and reignite your energy.

Know Your Numbers: When to Test

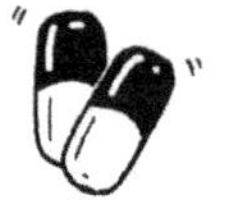

(Optional Tests to Discuss with Your GP or Practitioner)

- **DEXA Bone Scan** - Especially if you're at risk of osteoporosis.

- **Vitamin D, magnesium, and calcium levels** - All vital for bone and joint health.

- **Inflammatory markers** - If joint pain is a major issue.

Some practitioners (including myself) offer easy home test kits through consultation.

TCM Insight: The Organ Wisdom Behind Your Strength

In Traditional Chinese Medicine, movement is not just physical, it's energetic. Your body's ability to move smoothly and pain-free depends on several organ systems working in harmony:

- **Kidneys**: Govern bones, vitality, and stamina. Think of them as your body's power banks. If depleted, bones weaken and fatigue kicks in.

- **Liver**: Controls the smooth flow of blood and energy. If stuck (often due to stress), it can cause tightness, stiffness, or emotional frustration.

- **Spleen**: Supports muscle tone and digestion. Weak spleen energy = sluggish muscles, water retention, and bloating that affects how you move.

- **Lungs**: Nourish the skin and support oxygen flow which is key for circulation during physical activity.

TCM takeaway: When these organs are supported, movement becomes natural, healing, and energising, not exhausting.

Additional Insight - Movement is Medicine

I see it every day in my clinic. Women think that they're too tired to move, but in reality, they're stagnant and movement creates energy.

Start with five minutes. Walk the block. Squat while brushing your teeth. Stretch while the kettle boils.

Your body remembers how to move and it will thank you for it.

Want a structured strength plan that supports PeriMenopause without burnout? Email me directly and I'll send over my personal routine.

The Press-Pulsate-Pause Method™ for Strength, Joints & Bones

(Refer to Chapter 3 for full instructions)

Advanced Acupressure to Keep You Moving with Ease. You can use one point at a time, all at once, one side or both - whatever feels right. But remember: less is more.

- **Gallbladder 34 阳陵泉 (Yáng Líng Quán)**

    - You'll find this point on the outer side of your lower leg, just below the knee. Feel for a small dip in the muscle, slightly in front of the bony bump (fibula) on the outside of your leg. It's usually tender to the touch - a good sign you're in the right spot.

- Improves flexibility, relieves stiffness, and supports tendons and joint mobility.

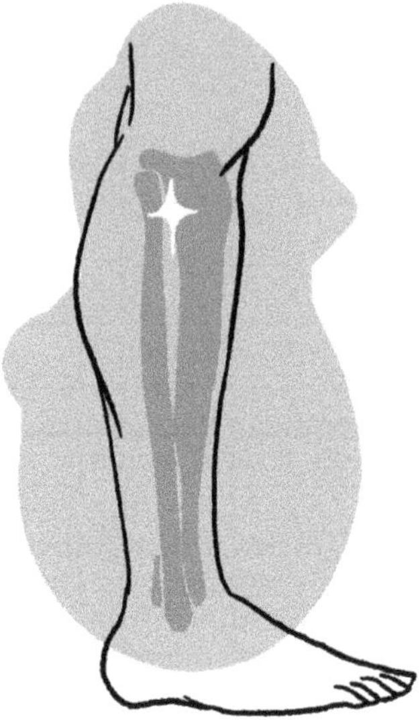

- **Kidney 3 太溪 (Tài Xī)**
    - Inside ankle, between the Achilles tendon and ankle bone.
    - Strengthens kidney energy, improves bone resilience, and supports your core vitality.

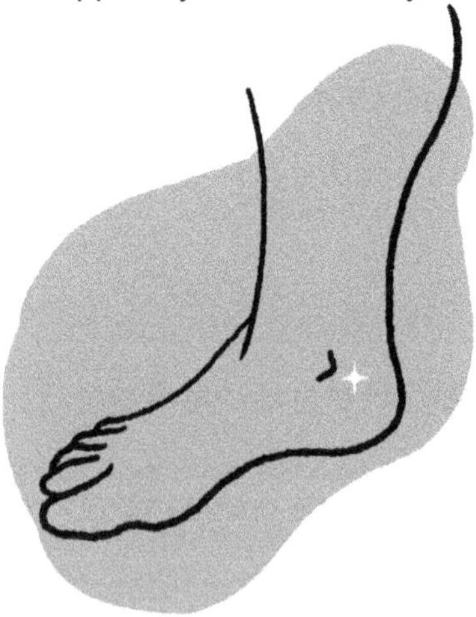

- **Stomach 36 足三里 (Zú Sān Lǐ)**
    - Four finger-widths below the kneecap, one finger-width to the outside of your shin bone.
    - Boosts energy, supports nutrient absorption, and aids physical recovery.

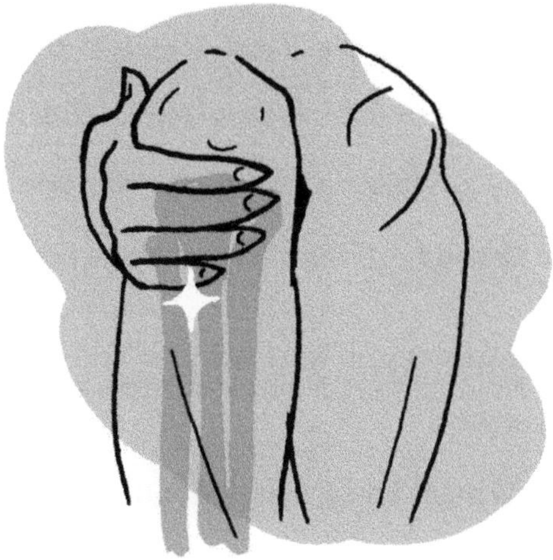

- **Liver 3 太冲 (Tài Chōng)**
    - Top of the foot, between big toe and second toe.
    - Eases tightness, promotes smooth flow, and calms emotional tension stored in the body.

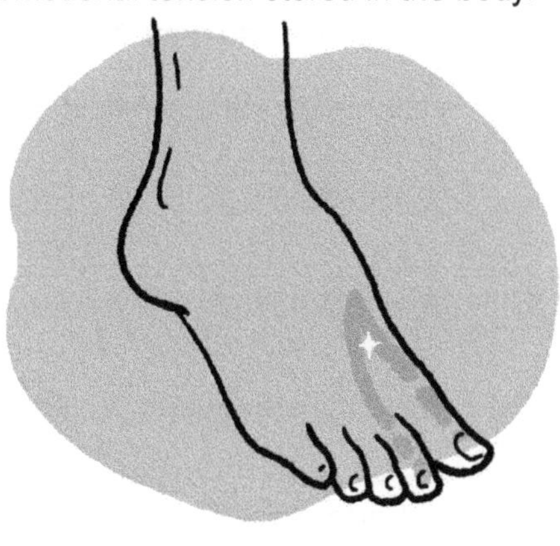

AromaAcu Therapy™ for Joint Ease & Movement Motivation

(Refer to Chapter 3 for how to use oils safely)

To reduce inflammation, stiffness, and emotional resistance to movement.

Recommended oils:

- **Ginger** - Warming and circulation-boosting; ideal for stiff joints.
- **Frankincense** - Anti-inflammatory and grounding.
- **Peppermint** - Invigorating, clears brain fog, and eases aches.
- **Lemon or Orange** - Uplifts mood, great for pre-workout motivation.

AcuWarrior™ Tip: Apply to your wrist (secured with a soft band if needed), inhale deeply during your acupressure practice, or place beside your mat during stretching.

Healing Breath Ritual to Ground & Glide

Ritual steps:

- Sit or stand comfortably with feet grounded.
- Inhale slowly through the nose, sending breath down through the hips, knees, and into the feet.
- Exhale, imagining tension melting from the joints.
- Affirm: "My body is strong, my joints are fluid, and I move through life with ease."

Quick Wins

- Warm your joints before activity. Use a heat pack or warm towel on knees/hips before walking or stretching.
- Walk daily - Even 10-15 minutes keeps circulation flowing and supports bones.
- Try a free YouTube stretch class. Search "gentle yoga for joints"

or “peri-safe strength workouts.” I know of a good online Strength Training programme. Feel free to email me for more info.

- Practice micro-movements such as squats while brushing teeth, calf raises while waiting for tea.
- Sip on turmeric tea or Sahar’s Chai™ which both support joint health. Check with your healthcare provider if you’re on medication.
- Consider collagen, magnesium, and vitamin D. They’re your bone and muscle allies. Speak to a health professional or book a supplement consultation with me.

Affirmation

“Every move I make builds my strength, supports my health, and empowers my journey through life.”

Gratitude Prompt

What did movement look like for me this week and how did it make me feel? Was it a stretch, a walk, a dance in the kitchen? Celebrate one moment your body showed up for you, no matter how small.Then ask: How can I honour this body again tomorrow?

Even on still days, your body is working for you. Let this be a moment of thanks.

Persian Wisdom

“The oak tree doesn’t compare itself to the willow; both stand strong in their own way.”

بلوط خود را با بید مقایسه نمی‌کند؛ هر دو به روش خود قوی‌اند

Transliteration: Balut khod râ bâ bid moghâyesé nemikonad; har do be ravesh-e khod ghavi-and.

Meaning: Your strength is personal. You don’t need to move like anyone else. Honour your way, your rhythm, your growth.

***Let's Keep Talking**: Share your movement wins with me using* **#PocketPeri** *and mention @AcuCareClinicUK. I'd love to hear how this chapter inspired you to move with more love, strength, or ease.*

***Next Up**: We're talking about something that nobody talks about enough: your sex drive.It's not just about hormones. It's about confidence, comfort, connection, and giving yourself permission to enjoy pleasure again.*

CHAPTER 15

Let's Talk About Sex, Baby

Reigniting Libido and Intimacy

Let's talk about something most women don't talk about, not honestly, anyway. If you've ever thought, "Where the hell did my libido go?" or "Why do I feel so disconnected from my body?" then you're not alone, and, no, there's nothing wrong with you.

Libido doesn't disappear in PeriMenopause but it does shapeshift. It may not look like it used to, but with the right support - emotionally, physically, hormonally - that spark can absolutely reignite. And when it does? It's not just about sex. It's about connection. Confidence. Sensual energy.

This chapter is your permission slip to explore it all, in your way, on your terms. And yes, we're going to say "Get your jiggy on!" because why not?

Western Insight - What's Really Happening to Your Libido

PeriMenopause doesn't cancel desire but it does complicate it. Here's the breakdown:

Hormonal Hijinks

- Oestrogen drops: This leads to vaginal dryness, reduced circulation, and sensitivity changes.
- Testosterone declines: This often-overlooked hormone plays a key role in libido and drive. When levels drop, so can your desire and your motivation to do anything about it.

Stress and Cortisol

When cortisol's high, desire's low. Stress physically blocks the body's ability to connect both emotionally and sexually.

Body Confidence Wobbles

Changing body shape, fluctuating weight (especially around the belly), and skin changes can make you feel 'meh', even if your partner still thinks you're hot!

TCM Insight: The Organs of Passion

In Traditional Chinese Medicine, libido isn't just hormonal. It's energetic, emotional, and constitutional. The main players?

- **Kidneys** - Store your vital energy and essence. Low kidney energy = low libido.
- **Liver** - Governs smooth emotional flow. When stressed or frustrated, it blocks arousal.
- **Spleen** - Your energy producer. If it's tired (from overwork, overthinking, or poor diet), everything else feels like a chore - including intimacy.

TCM Tip: Libido is like a garden and it needs nourishment, sunlight, and rest. Not just action.

The Shift: Redefining Desire

Desire isn't linear and it's not always spontaneous. But that doesn't mean it's gone. It just needs a different kind of invitation to the party.

Top Tips to Rekindle Your Spark:

1. **Date Yourself First** - Pleasure starts with self-care. Massage in jasmine or ylang ylang body oil after a warm shower. Light a candle. Touch your skin like you mean it.

2. **Communication Is Foreplay** - Awkward chats? Yes. Necessary? Also yes. Telling your partner what feels good (or what doesn't) can reignite connection.

3. **Rediscover Sensuality (Not Just Sex)** - Dancing in the kitchen. Long hugs. Hands on skin. Lying close with no agenda. This is intimacy.

4. **Use Tools Without Shame** - Moisturisers, lubes, oestrogen creams - they're practical solutions, not failures. Ask your GP, or speak to someone like me.

The Press-Pulsate-Pause Method™ for Sensual Energy

(Refer to Chapter 3 for full instructions)

These Advanced Acupressure points help restore sensual energy, circulation, and calm. You can use one point, or all - one side or both. Less is more.

- **Kidney 3 太溪 (Tài Xī)**
    - Inside ankle, between the Achilles tendon and ankle bone.
    - Boosts libido, energy, and vitality.

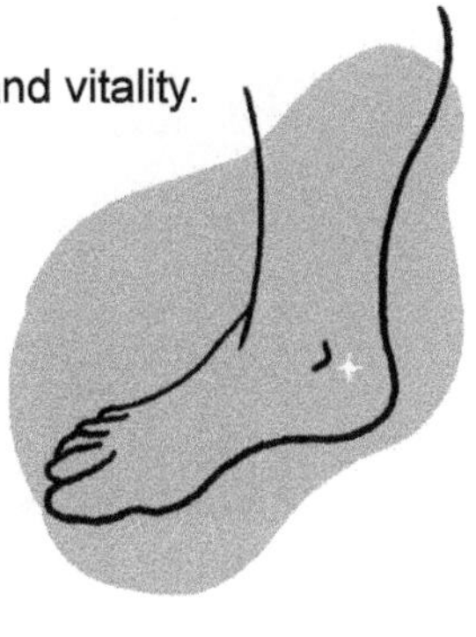

Fun Fact: I once did a demo video on this point and it went viral on TikTok. Thousands of views, with hilarious comments asking if it was my ankle or my underarm. (Spoiler: ankle, of course.)

- **Conception Vessel 4 (Ren 4) 关元 (Guān Yuán)**
    - Located four finger-widths directly below your belly button, in line with the centre of your body.
    - Revitalises sexual energy and hormonal harmony.
    - Avoid during pregnancy or if trying for a baby.

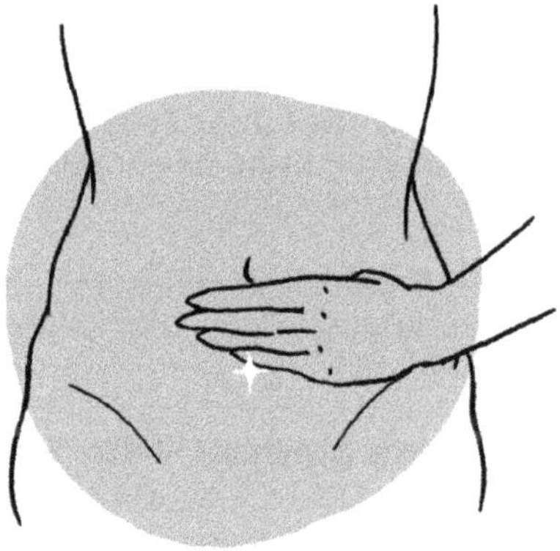

- **Liver 3 太冲 (Tài Chōng)**
    - Between the big toe and second toe (in the tender webbing).
    - Releases emotional tension and blocked desire.

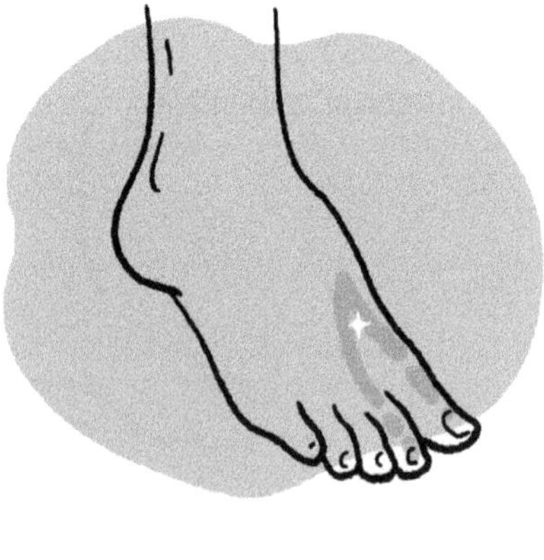

AromaAcu Therapy™ for Scents That Spark

(Refer to Chapter 3 for how to use oils safely)

Pair your acupressure with scent to awaken connection and calm.

Recommended oils:

- Ylang Ylang - Opens the heart and boosts sensual confidence.
- Jasmine - Euphoric and deeply connecting.
- Clary Sage - Relaxes the nervous system and balances hormones.
- Rose - Luxurious, loving, and perfect before a date night.

Healing Breath Ritual to Spark Passion

Ritual steps:

1. Lie down. One hand on your heart, the other on your lower abdomen.
2. Inhale slowly for 4 counts.
3. Hold for 2.
4. Exhale gently for 6.
5. Repeat 5-8 times.
6. Visualise: A golden warmth blooming in your lower belly, rising slowly through your pelvis, up to your chest and heart, grounding you, glowing within you, igniting your sensual spark.
7. Affirm: "I invite passion, joy, and connection into my life."

Quick Wins

- Rose tea before "jiggy-jiggy" - Soft, soothing, and opens the heart. Sip 30 minutes before and think of it as an inner love letter.
- Strong glutes, strong mojo. Strength training boosts blood flow, body confidence and, yes, bedroom stamina. Don't forget those

pelvic floor squeezes.

- Body oil rituals - Use post-shower oiling with slow, intentional touch. Not just skincare, it's self-connection.

- Collagen & Zinc - Your Undercover Confidence Boosters. As oestrogen dips, collagen levels follow which doesn't just affect your skin, but also the elasticity of your vaginal tissue and pelvic floor. Collagen can support both comfort and confidence, especially during intimacy. Zinc might not sound sexy, but it's a small-but-mighty mineral that helps with hormone production, mood stability, and even testosterone support - the hormone that gives your libido a lift. Both can make a subtle but powerful difference. If you're on medication or unsure what your body needs, always check first - or you're welcome to book a supplement consultation with me.

- The "No Pressure" rule - Not every cuddle has to lead somewhere but it's funny how often they do when there's no pressure.

- Remember the brain is the biggest sex organ - Read a spicy novel. Have a flirty daydream. That counts too.

Affirmation

"My desires are vibrant, my body is beautiful, and intimacy is a joyful connection to myself and those I love."

Gratitude Prompt

What's one thing I appreciated about my body or my sensuality this week?

It might be a moment of softness, a spark of desire, or simply choosing to reconnect in thought, touch, or presence. This isn't about performing. It's about permission.

Take a deep breath and thank your body for being yours.

Persian Wisdom

"Love starts within. When you honour yourself, intimacy becomes a celebration of who you are."

عشق از درون آغاز می‌شود. وقتی خودت را گرامی می‌داری، صمیمیت جشن وجود توست.

Transliteration: Eshgh az daroon āghāz mishavad. Vaghti khodet rā gerāmi midāri, samimiyat jashn-e vojud-e tost.

Meaning: Self-love is the root of sensual joy. Honour yourself, and connection becomes effortless.

***Let's Keep Talking**: Sex isn't a taboo here. It's a conversation. Tag me using* **#PocketPeri** *and mention @AcuCareClinicUK. I'd love to know which part of this chapter helped you feel seen, soothed, or a little more sexy.*

***Next Up**: I wanted to make sure this book truly gives you achievable self-care tools that help from the inside out. Let's talk collagen, glow, and grace without the anti-ageing nonsense.*

CHAPTER 16

Feel Good to Look Good

The Ultimate Guide to Radiant Skin During PeriMenopause

One-third of UK women are in PeriMenopause or menopause and their skin feels it too.

Let's be honest you can spend hundreds on skincare, but if your stress is sky-high, hormones are in chaos, and your sleep is in shambles then it'll still show on your face.

This chapter isn't just about skincare. It's about shifting the narrative. Most beauty advice tells us to "look good to feel good." But what if it's the other way around?

Let's flip the script. Forget the pressure to 'anti-age', we're here to 'pro-age'. Because as I always say "When you feel good, you look good. And when you look good, guess what? You feel even better."

It's a beautiful loop. And it starts with healing from the inside out. Not masking or fixing, but supporting your skin, hormones, and emotions like the teammates they are. Let's step into it.

Western Insight: The Hormone-Skin Collision

PeriMenopause is like your skin's mood swing phase. As oestrogen declines, so does collagen, the protein that keeps your skin plump, firm, and smooth. In fact, from around age 25, collagen production starts to decline. By PeriMenopause, it may decrease by up to 30%.

This doesn't just affect your skin. It impacts your joints, bones, and even muscle tone. Couple that with a drop in natural oils, slower cell turnover, and fluctuating hormones, and you may notice:

- Dryness.
- Sagging.
- Fine lines.
- Skin that feels more reactive or sensitive.
- And yes, acne and breakouts - just when you thought you'd left those in your teenage years.

TCM Insight: Your Skin is a Reflection of What's Within

Traditional Chinese Medicine (TCM) views the face as a map or a mirror reflecting what's happening in your internal organs and emotional landscape. Here's how your organ systems affect your glow:

Lungs and Sadness: Dull Skin, Loss of Self

In TCM, the Lungs govern the skin and are strongly linked to grief, but sometimes the grief isn't about loss but rather losing yourself. That subtle sadness of no longer recognising who you see in the mirror. "I just don't feel like myself anymore." Sound familiar?

Mini Ritual: Breathe Your Glow Back

Try this twice a day to re-energise your skin and your sense of self.

1. Place both hands on your lower ribs.
2. Inhale deeply for 4 counts and feel your ribs expand.
3. Hold for 4 and visualise fresh oxygen flowing to your skin cells.
4. Exhale slowly for 6 and let go of that low-grade emotional fog.

AcuWarrior™ Tip: Imagine each breath as a sunrise washing over your face.

Liver and Anger: Breakouts & Redness

Anger, frustration, and repressed rage overwork the Liver. That shows up on your forehead and cheeks as breakouts, irritation, or redness. Rage is a skin saboteur.

Try this: Place your hand under the lower right ribs (over your liver) while doing calming breathwork. Imagine the anger dissolving into thin air.

Kidneys and Fear: Puffiness, Tired Skin

Your Kidneys are your body's battery. They rule over hydration, vitality, and aging. When they're depleted by fear, stress, or overwork, the skin can look puffy, pale, or tired.

Recharging Ritual:

1. Place a warm compress or hot water bottle on your lower back each evening.
2. Do this while relaxing, feet up, hot cup of Sahar's Chai™ in hand.
3. Let your kidneys rest and reset.

AcuWarrior™ Tip: Rest isn't lazy, it's your secret beauty hack.

The Lookism Trap

From subtle ageist remarks to overt pressure to "stay young," lookism is real, especially at the workplace. This cultural obsession with appearing flawless affects women deeply throughout life, but even more during PeriMenopause, when natural changes can trigger self-doubt. Your worth is not in your wrinkles or how "tight" your skin is. It's in your wisdom, humour, experience, and radiant authenticity.

Remember: Every birthday is a privilege. A reminder that you're here, alive, and evolving. You've earned every line, every laugh, every lesson. Here's to another year of radiating beauty through wisdom and lived experience.

The Press-Pulsate-Pause Method™ for Skin Vitality

(See Chapter 3 for full instructions)

Use one point, or all four. One side or both. Whatever feels right but remember: less is more.

- **Stomach 36 足三里 (Zú Sān Lǐ)**
    - Four finger-widths below the kneecap, one finger-width to the outside of your shin bone.
    - More than just an energy booster, this point feeds your skin from the inside out. It kickstarts healthy blood flow, supports digestion (hello, nutrient absorption!), and delivers nourishment where your skin needs it most. Think of it as your skin's secret source of inner glow.

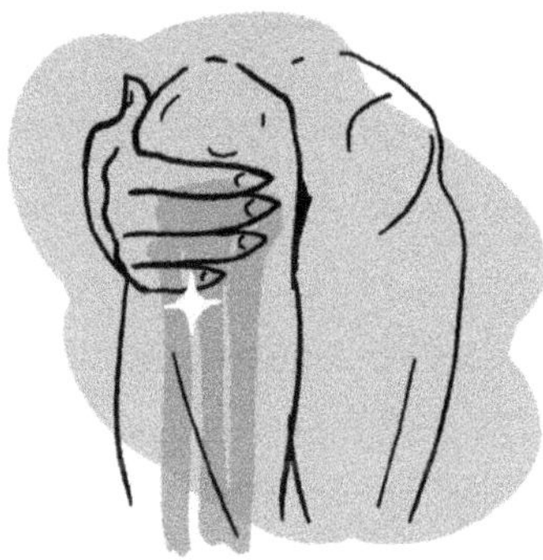

- **Large Intestine 11 曲池 (Qū Chí)**
    - At the outer end of your elbow crease (outer side), when your arm is bent.
    - This is your skin's Pressure Release Valve. Think of this point as a steam valve for your system helping to release internal heat, calm fiery flare-ups, and support your skin's natural detox flow. Perfect for when your skin's saying "I need out!" but your body's holding it in.

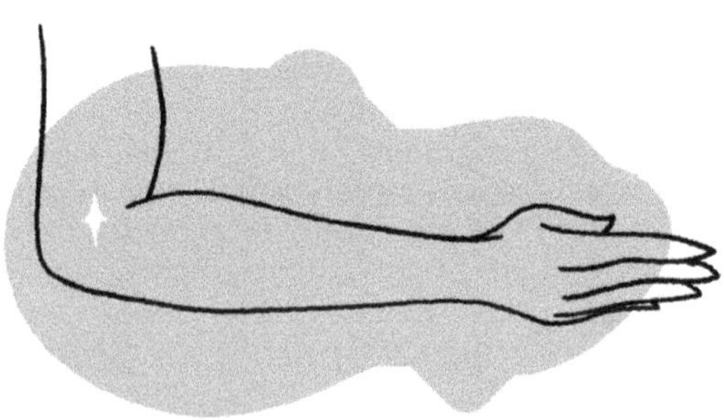

- **Kidney 3 太溪 (Tài Xī)**
    - Inside ankle, between the Achilles tendon and ankle bone.
    - This point taps into your body's inner reservoir - helping to replenish skin moisture, support elasticity, and restore that plump, nourished glow from within. When your skin feels tired or dry, Kidney 3 reminds it how to drink deeply again.

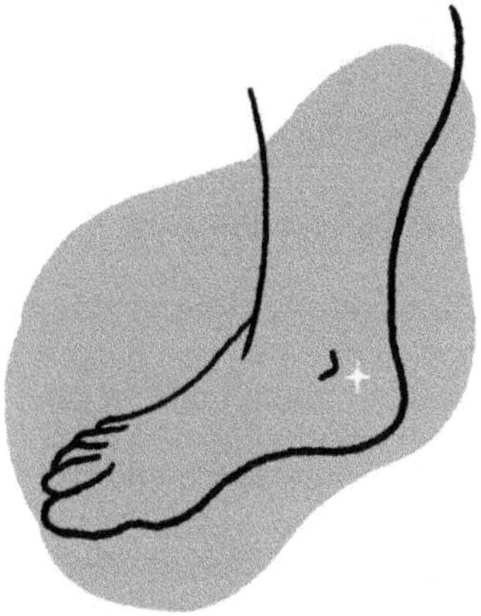

- **Liver 3 太冲 (Tài Chōng)**
    - Between the big toe and second toe (in the tender webbing).
    - This is your skin's reset button. It helps calm internal tension that often shows up on your skin, especially linked to emotions, hormones, or nervous system overload. Think of it as pressing reset when your skin and mood are on edge.

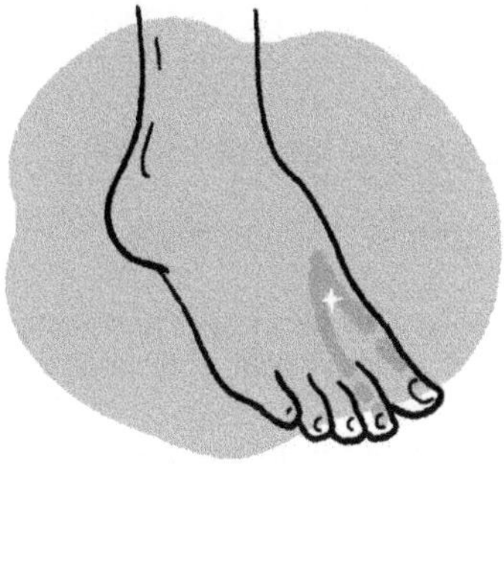

AcuWarrior™ Reminder: "Two minutes a day keeps the peri face at bay!"

AromaAcu Therapy™ for Radiant Skin

(Refer to Chapter 3 for how to use oils safely)

Recommended oils:

- Rose - Hydrates and uplifts mood. A timeless skin ally and a Persian favourite!
- Frankincense - Cellular rejuvenation and skin tone.
- Chamomile - Calms reactive skin.
- Geranium - Balances sebum and boosts circulation.

Craving skincare that actually understands your skin? Book a personalised consultation with me and I'll craft a bespoke blend that supports your skin from the outside in, and the inside out.

Collagen & Supplements: What You Need to Know

As mentioned previously, from your mid-20s, collagen begins to decline. By PeriMenopause, you could lose up to 30% affecting skin, joints, and more.

Types of Collagen:

- Type I: Skin, bones, tendons.
- Type II: Cartilage.
- Type III: Skin, muscles, vessels.

What to Look For:

- Hydrolysed collagen (for best absorption).
- Combine with Vitamin C for synthesis.
- Zinc: Supports wound healing and hormone balance (Short-term use recommended, always ask your practitioner).

I support patients across the globe, in clinic and online, and you're welcome to book a consultation with me for supplement advice that's personalised to your unique needs.

Let's Talk About Alcohol, Smoking & Drugs

These habits can wreak havoc on your skin and your hormones.

- Alcohol - Dehydrates, dulls the skin, disrupts sleep.
- Smoking - Reduces circulation, speeds up ageing, weakens collagen.
- Recreational drugs - Stress the liver and nervous system, often showing up on your face.

No shame here, just awareness. Your skin can't detox what you keep topping up.

The Bonus You Didn't Know You Needed: Facial Gua Sha + Your Own DIY Ritual

If you love rituals, this one's for you. Let this be your new bedtime favourite. A moment to wind down, tune in, and love on your skin like she's been waiting all day for this.

Block out a moment for you, once or twice a week. Evenings are ideal. Let the oils work their magic overnight while you drift into a deeper beauty sleep (yes, it's a thing).

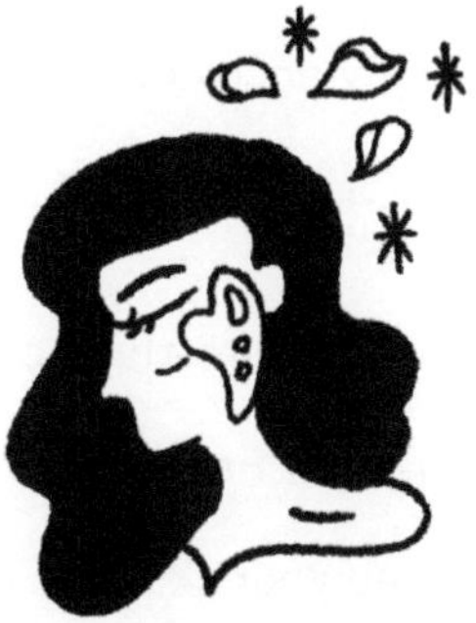

You'll need:

- 1 tsp jojoba oil.
- 1 drop of rose essential oil.

Warm a few drops between your palms, then glide from the centre of your face outward.

Use your Gua Sha stone or just your hands (you're allowed) and sweep with slow, upward, strokes. Aim for 2-5 strokes per area, repeating each section a few times over about 5 minutes.

This isn't skincare. This is a ritual. A mini rebellion against the rush. A moment of calm carved out just for you. Because your face deserves more than a quick rinse and go. It deserves presence. Intention. And a little love. I also stock beauty tools and oils. If you can't find them on the website, email me!

Healing Breath Ritual for a Glow from Within

Ritual steps:

1. Place one hand on your chest, and one on your belly.
2. Inhale for 4.
3. Hold for 4.
4. Exhale for 6.
5. Visualisation: Oxygen nourishing your skin like sunlight through your bloodstream.
6. Mantra: "With each breath, I nourish my skin from within."

Quick Wins

- Stay hydrated - Think water, cucumber, watermelon.
- Enjoy antioxidant-rich foods - Berries, leafy greens, green tea.
- Try Sahar's Chai™ or any other decaffeinated herbal tea instead of coffee.
- Do light stretching or a mini walk post-meal.
- Practice Facial Gua Sha routine 2x/week.
- Keep your skincare routine gentle and simple, not overloaded.
- Sleep! Your skin regenerates overnight.

Affirmation

"My skin is a reflection of my journey, unique and beautiful. I care for it with love and gratitude."

Gratitude Prompt

What's one way your skin showed up for you this week, even if it wasn't "perfect"? A glow after a walk, the softness of your cheeks, the warmth of a smile in the mirror? Take a moment to thank your skin. Not just for how it looks, but for how it protects, senses, and reflects your inner world.

This is where self-care becomes self-celebration.

Persian Wisdom

"Beauty is everywhe زیبایی همه جا هست، فقط گاهی لازم است در باغ قدم بزنیم تا آن را ببینیم.
see it." - Rumi

Transliteration: Zībāyi hamejā hast, faghat gāhi lāzem ast dar bāgh ghadam bezanim tā ān rā bebinim.

Meaning: Sometimes, beauty is closer than you think. It just needs your presence.

From One Queen to Another:

I asked my incredible mother, Parvin, to share some Persian wisdom with us all:

"Each stage of life brings secret goodies, even if they're hiding."

It's a Persian truth I now live by. Ageing is a wild, beautiful adventure, not a curse. Let's normalise being pro-age, not anti-age.

Let's Keep Talking: *Tag me using* **#PocketPeri** *and mention @AcuCareClinicUK. I'd love to hear how this chapter shifted the way you think about beauty and skin. Let's reclaim your glow on your own terms.*

Next Up: *We're switching it up! Think of this next chapter like your kitchen junk drawer… if that drawer happened to be full of hormone hacks, skin tricks, and random-but-genius tips that actually make life easier.*

@ACUCARE_CLINIC_UK

CHAPTER 17

Scattered Gems

Welcome to Your Peri Drawer

Not everything has to be a full protocol or major revelation. Sometimes it's the small, oddly specific things that get you through the week. The kind of hacks that don't need an individual chapter, but deserve a place in your life.

Think of this chapter as THAT kitchen drawer. You know the one filled with random bits and bobs. The safety pins, loose batteries, birthday candles, maybe a rogue herbal tea bag. It might look chaotic, but everything in there has value. This is your Peri Drawer - full of little gems to make your days smoother, brighter, and a little more *'you.'*

What's Inside the Drawer?

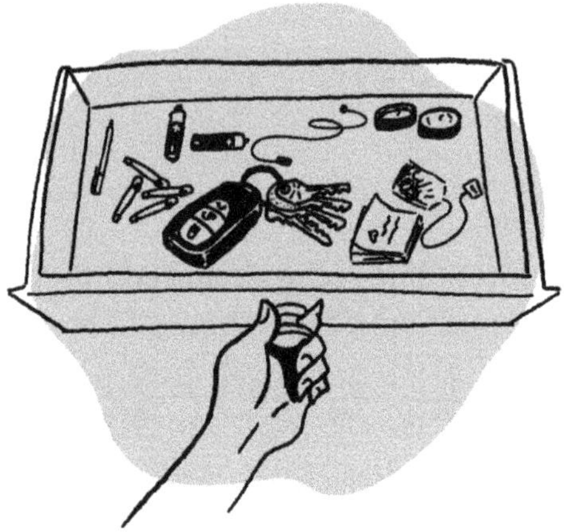

Why Do I Feel So Scattered?

Losing track of your thoughts mid-sentence? Constantly distracted, even during things you want to do? Welcome to the brain-fuzz zone of PeriMenopause. So what's really going on?

When oestrogen drops, so does dopamine - a neurotransmitter (chemical messenger) responsible for focus, motivation, and mental clarity. Add in poor sleep, inflammation, emotional load, and boom, your brain feels scrambled.

Sometimes it's just a phase of hormonal chaos. But for some, this scattered feeling may also flag up traits of ADHD, especially in women whose symptoms were missed in childhood.

Mini self-check (Not a diagnosis!). Tick what applies to you most days:

- □ I forget what I was doing mid-task.
- □ I leave cupboards open without realising.
- □ I interrupt or talk over people.
- □ I struggle to follow long conversations or instructions.
- □ I'm constantly misplacing things (keys, phone, mind).
- □ My mind races at bedtime even if I'm exhausted.

If you tick several, it's worth exploring further. ADHD in women often goes undiagnosed until later life. If this sounds familiar, speak to a qualified specialist or you're welcome to book a complimentary initial consultation with me to explore what's next.**

Do I Have to Wear Makeup?

Not unless you want to. This is about choice, not obligation. Makeup can feel empowering, creative, and fun but it can also become a quiet pressure, especially when your skin isn't "behaving."

Here's the thing: Any skin symptom is a message. A gentle (or not-so-gentle) nudge from your body saying something deeper needs support. Whether it's dryness, dullness, acne, or puffiness. It's not just about your skincare routine. It's about internal nourishment and healing.

And yes, I get it. I had adult acne in my mid-twenties. It was tough to even imagine not wearing foundation back then. But that was before I became an acupuncture practitioner. Since then, I've experimented with going makeup-free for seven years, and it's been unexpectedly liberating. I'll go deeper into that story in my next book. But for now, here's a gentle challenge:

Try going bare-faced once a week. Not to "be brave" but to give your face space to breathe. Feeling hesitant? That's okay. See this as an experiment, not a punishment. And if you don't feel comfortable going bare-faced that's absolutely fine. We don't need to add more stress to the situation.

If you try it, tag me using **#PocketPeri** and mention @AcuCareClinicUK. I love hearing how small experiments like this can make a big difference.

When Anxiety Sneaks In

Hormonal changes can dial up your nervous system without warning. One minute you're fine, the next, you're sweating the small stuff (or everything).

Simple grounding trick: Place one hand over your belly. Inhale slowly and feel your hand rise. Exhale and feel it fall. Belly breathing activates the vagus nerve which is a direct line to your calm response.

Scan the QR code to access my "De-Stress in Three Steps" method. It's a great place to start when everything feels like too much.

Itchy Ears? You're Not Imagining It!

Suddenly scratching at your ears more than usual? This little-discussed symptom is surprisingly common during PeriMenopause. Why? Declining oestrogen dries out the body's tissues, including your ear canal area, which can become sensitive or reactive to new allergens.

You might also notice:

- Random skin flare-ups.
- Itching in unusual places.
- A new wave of allergies (yep, even in your 40s).

Try this:

1. Apply a tiny bit of warm, fragrance-free oil (like olive or almond) around the entrance of your ear. Don't apply it inside.
2. Gently cup your hands over your ears and press lightly. I sometimes find this relieves the pressure for a moment.

This is a symptom I personally struggled with, and still occasionally do. It's underrated but manageable with the right guidance. In the meantime, if this sounds familiar then it's worth checking for common culprits like allergies or even something as simple as earwax build-up.

Why does my scalp feel like something is crawling on it?

Random tingles, prickles, or that "there's something on my skin" feeling? You're not losing it! This is another under-talked-about PeriMenopause quirk.

Declining oestrogen and progesterone affect nerve endings and skin sensitivity. Combine that with stress and hormonal shifts, and your scalp and skin can send some seriously confusing signals.

Pro Tip: Resist the urge to scratch like mad! Instead try a gentle scalp massage with your fingertips or a soft brush to calm nerve endings and improve circulation.

AromaAcu Therapy™:A drop of chamomile or lavender on a damp cotton pad inhaled deeply can soothe the nervous system from the inside out. (See Chapter 3 for how to use oils safely)

The Press-Pulsate-Pause Method™: (Refer to Chapter 3 for full instructions)

- **Large Intestine 11 曲池 (Qū Chí)**
    - At the outer crease of your bent elbow.
    - Known for calming irritation and supporting skin balance.

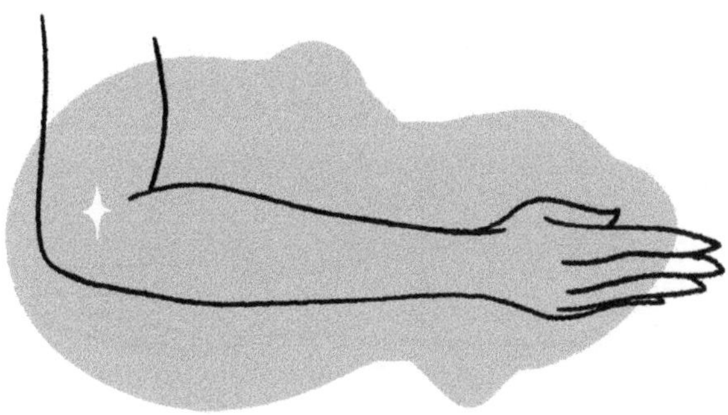

AcuWarrior™ Tip: If you notice persistent dryness, flaking, or irritation on your scalp or skin, don't just layer on more products. Sometimes it's as simple as an allergy, a bit of build-up, or even a mild fungal infection triggered by excess sweating from night sweats or scalp perspiration. Get a proper assessment if you suspect dandruff, sensitivity, or fungal overgrowth. Self-care starts with smart care and that includes knowing when to get professional eyes on it.

Has your scalp ever tricked you into thinking something's crawling there? Tag me using **#PocketPeri** and mention @AcuCareClinicUK. Let's normalise these "wait, is this just me?" moments.

Acupuncture: Your Natural Antihistamine

Forget drowsy pills. Traditional acupuncture can be an effective way to manage inflammation, itchiness, and allergy-like symptoms. Need a go-to for your self-care stash? This Advanced Acupressure point is one of my all-time favourites:

The Press-Pulsate-Pause Method™: (Refer to Chapter 3 for full instructions)

- **Large Intestine 11 曲池 (Qū Chí)**
    - At the outer end of your elbow crease (outer side), when your arm is bent.
    - Use this point when allergies flare or you feel inflamed.
    - Hold for up to 2 minutes with steady, calming breaths.

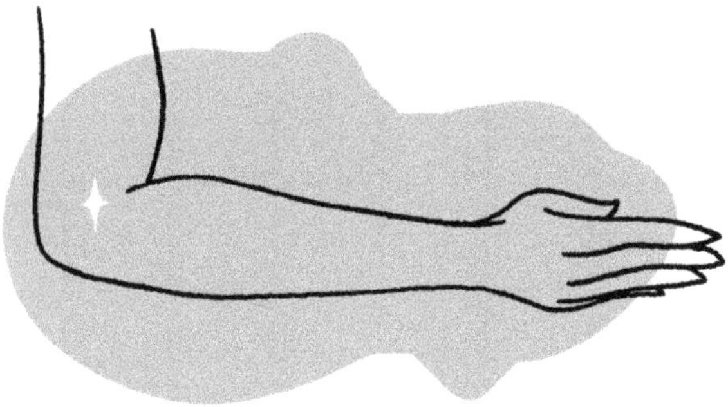

Feeling Puffy and Puffy and… Puffy?

Water retention during PeriMenopause is real and relentless.

Lower oestrogen can affect your kidneys, circulation, and lymphatic system, making it harder for your body to shift fluids. That's why some mornings you wake up with swollen fingers, puffy eyes, or ankles that feel twice their size. You're not imagining it. You're inflamed, not "fat."

- Hydrate smart. Sipping warm water (yes, warm) supports kidney function and reduces internal stress on your digestive system.

- Lymph-supporting teas like dandelion, nettle, or parsley can gently encourage drainage. (Sahar's Chai™ includes cinnamon and ginger, and see Chapter 12 for more gut/puffiness insight.)

- Gua Sha tool or tapping massage: Use your Gua Sha tool gently along the cheekbones and under the eyes, sweeping outward towards your ears. Or, simply use your fingertips to tap around this area to stimulate lymphatic flow.

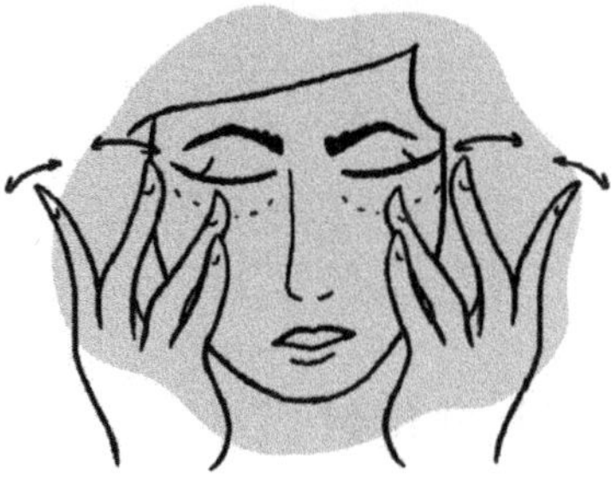

- Try dry body brushing before your morning shower. Always brush upwards towards your heart to boost circulation and lymph flow.

The Press-Pulsate-Pause Method™: (Refer to Chapter 3 for full instructions)

- **Spleen 9 阴陵泉 (Yīn Líng Quán)**
    - On the inner side of the lower leg, just below the knee crease, in a soft hollow.
    - Use this point to support water metabolism and ease puffiness.
    - Hold for up to 2 minutes on each side while breathing slowly.

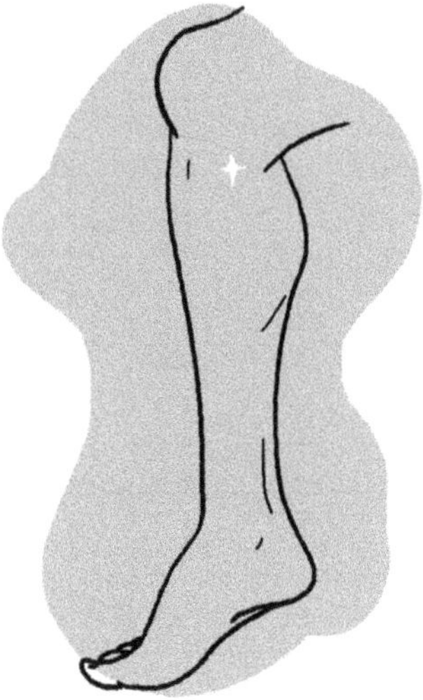

Craving Salty Snacks at Night?

It's not just comfort eating. Craving salty foods could be your Kidneys calling out for support.

In Traditional Chinese Medicine, salt is the flavour linked to the Kidneys the organ system responsible for your deepest reserves of energy, hormone balance, and bone strength. During PeriMenopause, the Kidneys are working overtime to keep things stable, especially when stress, sleep deprivation, or burnout creep in. And when they're running low? They shout and it often sounds like crisps, cheese, or salted nuts.

Try this instead:

- A pinch of natural sea salt to warm water or soup. It can support mineral balance without the snack spiral.
- Include mineral-rich foods like seaweed, sesame seeds, miso, or dark leafy greens in your meals.

AromaAcu Therapy™: Apply 1 drop of frankincense or vetiver on damp cotton wool and place it near your bed (Refer to Chapter 3 for how to use oils safely).

Healing Breath Ritual for Kidneys

Ritual Steps:

1. Place both hands over your lower back (kidney area).

2. Inhale deeply, imagining calm, cooling energy flowing into this space.

3. Exhale slowly, visualising tension releasing down your legs into the ground.

4. Repeat 6-9 times before bed and your body will thank you.

Why am I crying at everything?

Tears at random TV ads? Sudden sadness at a song you've heard a hundred times? It's not you being "too sensitive". It's a real, hormonal shift. When oestrogen dips, it affects your brain's chemical messengers (neurotransmitters) especially serotonin and dopamine, which help regulate mood and stress. Add in exhaustion, overstimulation, and a world that never stops, and of course the tears come.

AcuWarrior™ Tip: Let the tears flow. You don't need to fix it, just let it move through you. Place one drop of rose or neroli on damp cotton wool and hold it near your chest while breathing deeply (Refer to Chapter 3 for how to use oils safely).

The Press-Pulsate-Pause Method™: (Refer to Chapter 3 for full instructions)

- **Heart 7 神门 (Shén Mén)**
  - On the wrist crease, in line with the pinky finger.

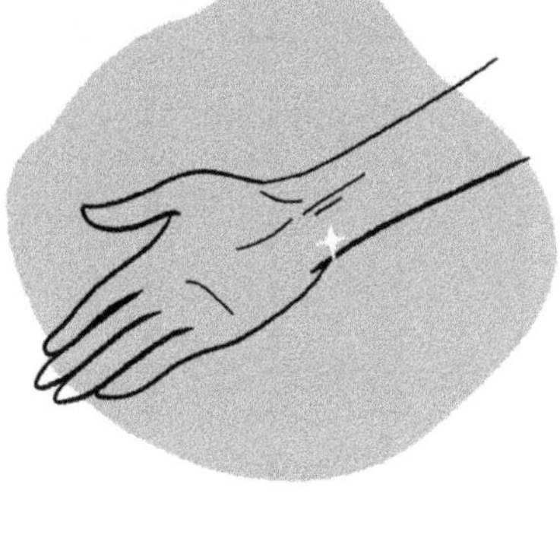

Been there? Tag me using **#PocketPeri** and mention @AcuCareClinicUK - and tell me your 'crying at a car advert' moment. I promise, you're not alone.

Reminder: Rest Isn't a Reward. It's a Reset. You don't have to earn your downtime. During PeriMenopause, rest becomes fuel and not a luxury. Your body is shifting, recalibrating, and calling for more softness, more repair and more grace.

Try this:

1. Switch to flight mode an hour before bed or, if you need to stay contactable, turn off notifications and only allow emergency calls (check your phone's "Do Not Disturb" settings).

2. Create a wind-down routine with calming essential oils like lavender, clary sage, or sweet orange, placed on damp cotton wool by your bed. (See Chapter 3 for how to use oils safely)

3. Read something nurturing. (Ahem... maybe this book.)

4. Remind yourself: "I deserve to rest - not just recover."

What if my GP doesn't get it?

PeriMenopause doesn't always show up clearly on blood tests, and many symptoms can be misread. But that doesn't mean you're making it up. It means the system still has catching up to do.

The truth? Some GPs get it. Some don't. And that's not your fault.

I got lucky. (Shout out to Dr Rem Lee!). He listened, and that made all the difference, but if you don't feel heard, keep going. Get a second opinion. Bring a symptom tracker (refer to Chapter 2). Be clear, assertive, and confident, not apologetic. You deserve care.

You can also book a 20-minute complimentary consultation with me online (UK time) or in person. Just an initial chat to understand what support you need. Sometimes that first step is everything.

Feeling Stuck? (A Quick Win for Bloating & Constipation)

Even though gut health has its own chapter, let's be real sometimes you just need a fast fix.

- Rub your tummy in gentle clockwise circles (it follows the direction of your colon).
- Sip warm water with lemon first thing in the morning.
- See Chapter 12 for the full gut reset.

The Press-Pulsate-Pause Method™: (Refer to Chapter 3 for full instructions)

- **Large Intestine 4 合谷 (Hé Gǔ).**
    - In the web between thumb and index finger.
    - Supports healthy bowel movement and helps things move along.

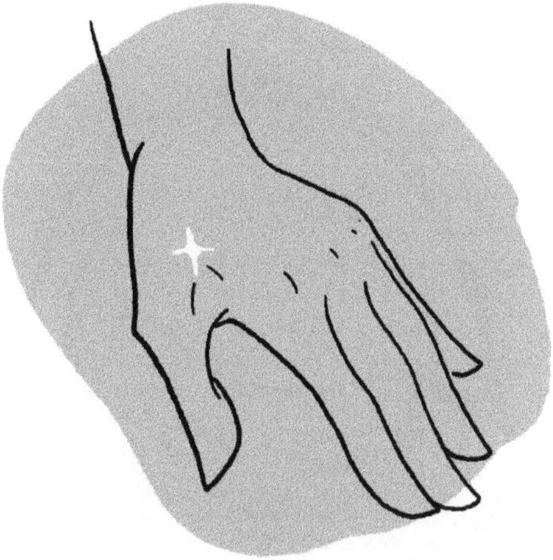

Bladder Wobbles & Pelvic Floor Blips

Let's talk leaks. Worried about laughing too hard? Afraid of unexpectedly sneezing? Suddenly bolting for the loo? "Stop and clench" your new mantra? (If you know, you know!)

You're not abnormal. You're in PeriMenopause and your pelvic floor is adjusting to the hormonal shift, especially as oestrogen levels begin to dip. It's incredibly common, and no, you don't just have to "live with it."

What helps:

- Do your pelvic floor exercises daily (yes, Kegels! Lift, hold, release).
- Focus on core-based movement like Pilates, yoga, or mindful breathwork.

The Press-Pulsate-Pause Method™: (Refer to Chapter 3 for full instructions)

- **DU20 百会 (Bǎi Huì)**
  - Crown of the head in line with the tips of your ears.
  - In TCM, this point helps lift your energy, support prolapse, and calm the nervous system.
  - Gently press this point for up to 2 minutes while breathing deeply.

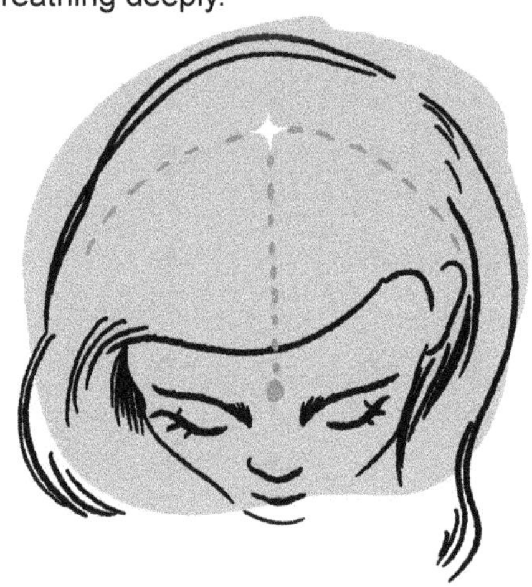

Speak to your GP first to rule out infections or anything requiring medical follow-up.

Then connect with a fully qualified Acupuncture Practitioner, preferably a member of the British Acupuncture Council (BAcC). Look for someone degree-trained and experienced in women's health. If you're looking for extra support, I offer both online consultations and in-person sessions at my clinic locations, tailored to help you navigate symptoms like bladder changes with clarity and confidence.

Scan here for booking link.

Caffeine Curfew: Your Nervous System Will Thank You

You've heard of beauty sleep, but have you met her nemesis? Her name's Caffeine. Caffeine stimulates your nervous system, which is great until it's 9 p.m. and your brain thinks it's hosting a TED Talk. During PeriMenopause, you may become more sensitive to caffeine, especially as oestrogen drops and adrenal load increases.

AcuWarrior™ Tip: No coffee, black tea, or matcha after 2pm. Swap for calming herbal teas like Sahar's Chai™, chamomile, or rooibos in the evening. Your sleep (and hormones) will thank you.

The Press-Pulsate-Pause Method™: (Refer to Chapter 3 for full instructions)

- **Heart 7 神门 (Shén Mén)**
    - On the wrist crease, in line with the pinky finger.

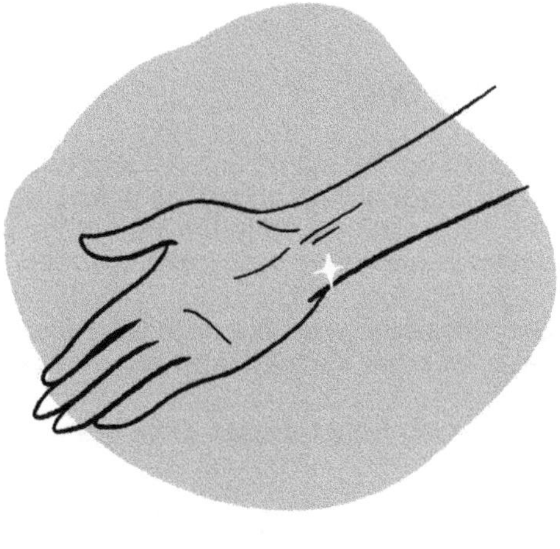

Pro Tip: Pair with a drop of clary sage or sweet orange on damp cotton wool (Refer to Chapter 3 for how to use oils safely).

You don't have to ditch coffee completely, just time it wisely.

Smoke, Sip… and Shift?

This isn't a lecture. Just a gentle reminder that alcohol and smoking can hit differently during PeriMenopause.

Your liver is already juggling hormone metabolism, and adding alcohol or tobacco to the mix can ramp up inflammation, disrupt your sleep, spike anxiety, and trigger hot flushes. What used to be a "glass to unwind" might now leave you wired at 3am or puffier the next morning.

Try this instead:

- Swap your evening drink for sparkling water with lime, or a calming blend like Sahar's Chai™ with cinnamon and ginger, to support digestion and warmth.
- If you smoke, be aware it can worsen symptoms like night sweats, itchy skin, and bone density loss.
- Craving a ritual? Light a natural soy-based candle, use your Gua Sha, or massage a calming oil onto your wrists instead - keep the ritual, change the tool.

The Press-Pulsate-Pause Method™: (Refer to Chapter 3 for full instructions)

- **Lung 7 列缺 (Liè Quē)**
    - Located on the thumb side of your wrist, about one and a half finger widths above the wrist crease. You'll find it in a slight dip, just off to the side of the bone. It's often easier to feel when your palm is turned towards you.
    - Use this point when the urge feels stronger than your calm, whether it's food, emotion, or overwhelm.
    - Hold gently for 2 minutes while breathing slowly and deeply.

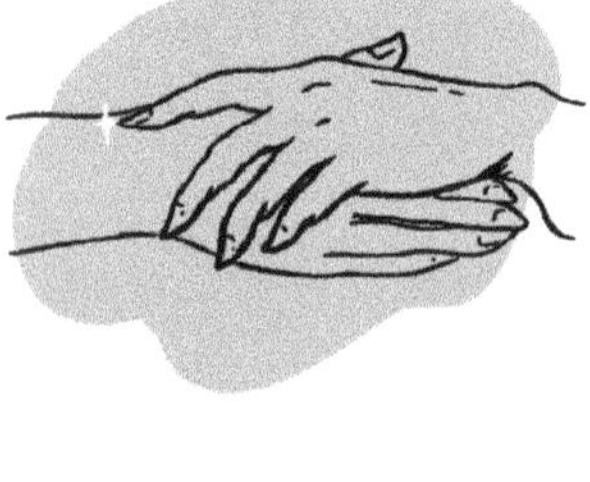

Let go of the urge, not your self-compassion. This is not about resisting or punishing yourself. It's about choosing calm without self-judgement.

AcuWarrior™ Tip: You're not being "bad", you're being human, but even a small shift can lead to big wins in sleep, energy, and hormone harmony.

The Toxic Candle Trap

You light it for calm but it might be lighting up chaos in your hormones.

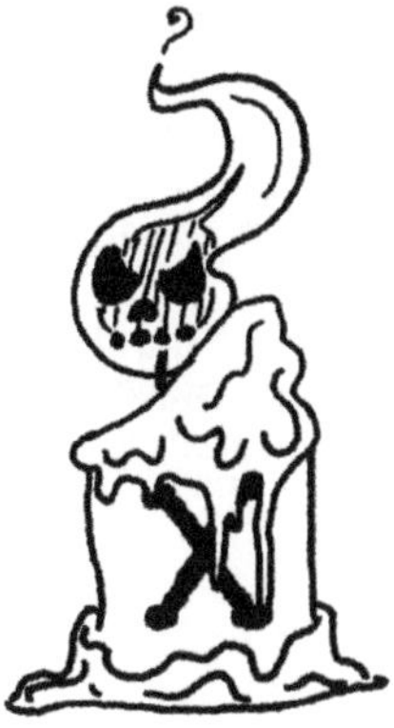

Paraffin wax and synthetic fragrance oils can release hormone-disrupting chemicals into the air. During PeriMenopause, your system is already juggling enough - no need for extra sabotage.

Swap Tip: Use soy-based or beeswax candles scented with pure essential oils (like lavender, geranium, or sweet orange) but always check ingredients. I've seen it firsthand: candles labelled as "soya-based" and "natural" but underneath all the earthy branding? Synthetic chemical fragrances. What a let-down...

AcuWarrior™ Tip: Candles are for ambiance, not hormone disruption. Read those labels like your health depends on it (because it does). Plus soy and beeswax are better for the environment too!

Perfume & Skincare Hormone Disruptors

That dreamy perfume bottle on your dresser? It might be a wolf in floral clothing.

Many high-street beauty products contain phthalates, parabens, and artificial fragrances. All known endocrine disruptors. These can mimic or block oestrogen, causing more hormonal mayhem.

What to avoid:

- Anything with "fragrance" as a vague ingredient.
- Products without full transparency on their labels.
- Overly scented body sprays, lotions, or oils.

AcuWarrior™ Tip: Your skin is your second mouth. Don't feed it toxic nonsense. Try DIY blends with rosehip oil, a single drop of pure rose, lavender, or frankincense. (Bonus: cheaper and customisable.) I've started making my own and I'm still experimenting to find my favourite that hits the spot!

I'm not here to tell you what to do, just to share my knowledge. Fragrance has an emotional element as well. If you love that branded scent because of memories associated with it or the way you feel when wearing it, then just think about how often and where you use it.

Who Am I? A Reflection with Kidney 23 神封 (Shén Fēng)

In Traditional Chinese Medicine, Kidney 23 is known as the Spirit Gate and is linked to your identity, confidence, and clarity. It's a brilliant point to use when you feel a little lost or unsure of who you're becoming.

Place your hand just below your collarbone and slide down to the space between your 4th and 5th ribs, about 2 finger-widths out from the centre of your chest, in line with the nipple (for most people). It sits just under the breast line, in that soft space between the ribs.

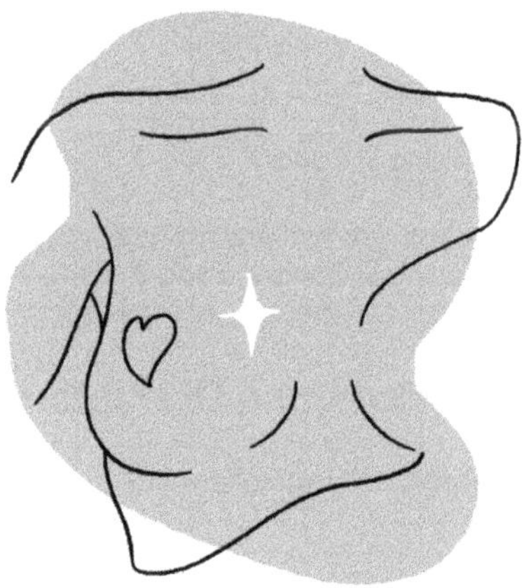

How to use:

Press gently with your fingertips while breathing slowly. As you do, ask yourself: "Who am I becoming in this new phase of life?" You don't need all the answers, just a moment to reconnect with yourself. This is more than acupressure. It's soul work.

Creepy Menopause Symptoms? You're Not Alone!

Seeing flickers or shadows that aren't there? Feeling like someone's watching when you're home alone? It sounds spooky but it's surprisingly common.

Hormonal shifts during PeriMenopause can heighten sensory awareness, distort perception, and even trigger mild visual hallucinations in rare cases (especially when you're sleep-deprived or overstimulated).

What to do:

- Get checked by your GP to rule out migraines, sleep disorders, or neurological causes.
- Practise grounding techniques:
    - Name three things you can see.
    - Two things you can touch.
    - One thing you can hear.

You're not going mad. You're recalibrating. Trust your body and ground your mind.

Hormone Confusion? Start Here.

If your moods, energy, or periods are suddenly all over the place, it could be PeriMenopause but don't assume this. If you're ready to understand what's really going on then:

Ask your GP about checking these key markers: Iron, Thyroid (TSH + T4), B12, and Vitamin D.

Prefer at-home testing and holistic guidance? I offer complimentary 20-minute consultations (UK time, online or in person) to help you explore your next step. No pressure, just clarity.

Mood Flip Trick

Bad mood brewing? Try this rebellious reset because mood swings deserve recognition, not shame.

The Press-Pulsate-Pause Method™: (Refer to Chapter 3 for full instructions)

- **Heart 7 神门 (Shén Mén)**
    - On the wrist crease, in line with the pinky finger.

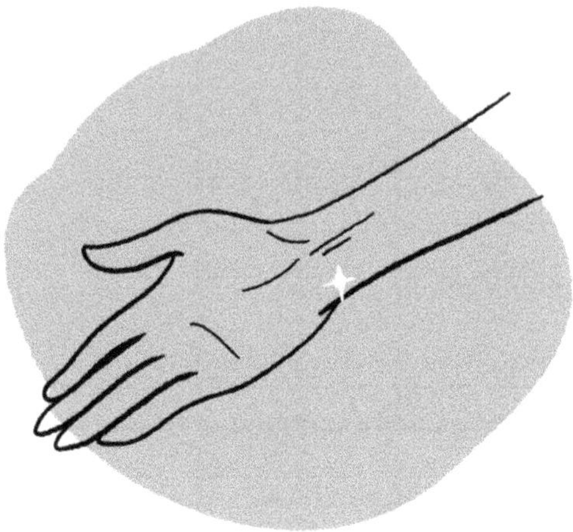

Also try this:

- Breathe slowly into your chest - in for four, out for six. Repeat.
- Blast your favourite 80/90s track (yes, at full volume).
- Dance like no one's judging, especially not your hormones.
- See Chapter 6 if your moods feel like a full-blown rollercoaster.

Something Special: Join our community playlist: PocketPeri - The Empowerment Mix on Spotify. It's a co-created space - submit your favourite tracks via @AcuCareClinicUK on Instagram. Because healing isn't just science, it's song, it's story, and it's shared space.

Feel united through the power of shared music!

A Final AcuWarrior™ Nudge

Let's close this drawer with a reminder worth tattooing on your soul: "You're not falling apart, you're reacalibrating."

Even if you only try one tool from this chapter, you're already showing up for yourself and that counts. PeriPower isn't about doing everything. It's about doing something consistently, compassionately, and in your own way.

AcuWarrior™ Reminder: "Two minutes a day keeps the peri away."

You're doing better than you think. You've absolutely got this.

Affirmation

"I honour the small wins. The little rituals. The scattered gems that bring me home to myself."

Gratitude Prompt

What's one "small but mighty" thing that supported you this week? Was it a soothing cup of tea, a playlist that lifted your mood, or remembering a tip from this book right when you needed it? Write it down. Celebrate the little things because they often make the biggest difference.

Your Peri Drawer is full of treasures. Don't underestimate their power.

Persian Wisdom

"Even a single thread can hold a jewel."

نخ نازک هم می‌تواند گنجی نگه دارد

Transliteration: Nakh-e nāzok ham mitavānad ganji negah dārad

Meaning: Small actions, tiny shifts, even seemingly insignificant rituals - they carry great value. Just like your Peri Drawer, life's hidden gems often come in the most humble forms.

Let's Keep Talking: *This drawer's always open. Tag your favourite gems, share your rituals, or just drop me a message if something lands. Tag us using* **#PocketPeri** *and mention @AcuCareClinicUK. I'd love to know which tip saved your day.*

Next Up: *Let's clear the fog and call out the fiction. We're unpacking the myths that keep women confused, dismissed, or doubting themselves from "you're too young" to "just take HRT and carry on."*

CHAPTER 18

Myth-Busting

Breaking Down the PeriMenopause Myths

Let's get one thing straight: PeriMenopause is already confusing enough without half-baked advice, well-meaning friends, or that one article you skimmed at 2am. This chapter is your myth-slaying space. We're calling out the outdated beliefs, hormonal half-truths, and flat-out nonsense that women are fed every day, especially when we're at our most vulnerable.

Because when you're informed, you're empowered. And when you're empowered, you can advocate, speak up, and make the decisions that serve your body best. Let's do this.

AcuWarrior™ Tip: Believing everything you hear is like taking directions from someone who's never been to your destination.

Let's set the record straight.

The Myths (and the Truths)

Myth #1: Menopause and PeriMenopause Are the Same Thing

The Myth: They're interchangeable terms.

The Reality: PeriMenopause is the hormonal build-up; menopause is defined as 12 consecutive months without a period. One's the road trip, the other's the destination.

Reminder: Don't blame menopause for everything. It hasn't even arrived yet.

Myth #2: You're Too Young for PeriMenopause

The Myth: PeriMenopause only starts after 50.

The Reality: Many women notice symptoms in their late 30s or early 40s. Mood swings, irregular periods, brain fog? They're waving flags.

Reminder: There's no "right" age. It's your body, your timeline.

Myth #3: Weight Gain Is Inevitable

The Myth: You'll gain weight no matter what.

The Reality: Hormones can shift how your body stores fat, but it's not inevitable. Movement, nutrition, and stress management matter more than ever.

Reminder: You're not at the mercy of your hormones. They work for you, not the other way around.

Myth #4: HRT Is Dangerous for Everyone

The Myth: HRT is a universal no-no.

The Reality: It's nuanced. HRT can be life-changing for some. This book focuses on natural approaches, but knowledge is power. Speak to a trusted health professional who understands your needs and risks.

Myth #5: Symptoms Are All in Your Head

The Myth: You're overreacting.

The Reality: Hot flushes, sleep disruption, mood changes, and more are real physiological events rooted in hormonal shifts.

Reminder: You're not imagining it and you're not alone.

Myth #6: PeriMenopause Means No More Sex Drive

The Myth: Libido disappears forever.

The Reality: Desire may dip, but it evolves and with the right support, it can return stronger than ever. Acupressure, aromatherapy, communication, and self-connection help.

Reminder: Passion doesn't pause. It gets smarter.

Myth #7: Sweating Is Just a Menopause Thing

The Myth: Night sweats only show up in menopause.

The Reality: Sweating can strike at any stage. It's often linked to oestrogen fluctuations, but not all women experience hot flushes.

Reminder: Keep a cooling mist, fan, or chilled pillow spray close. And no, it's not "just a hot day."

Myth #8: PeriMenopause Ends All Creativity

The Myth: Brain fog = game over.

The Reality: Creativity may dip with fatigue, but this is also a time of reinvention. Many women find their voice, clarity, or boldest work during PeriMenopause.

Reminder: This isn't the end, it's an edit. You're the author and you may even write a book!

HPV and PeriMenopause: Empowering Your Cervical Health

Let's bust some myths around HPV too because this one really matters.

Why It Matters

HPV isn't just for the young. With declining oestrogen and a slower immune response, dormant strains of HPV can reactivate during PeriMenopause. That makes regular screening, immune support, and education vital, not optional.

Myth-Busting: HPV Edition

Myth #1: You only get it if you sleep with multiple partners.

The myth: HPV means infidelity.

The reality: HPV can lie dormant for decades. A new diagnosis doesn't mean recent exposure.

Myth #2: Only young people can get it.

The myth: No need for cervical screenings after menopause.

The reality: Screening remains essential until at least 64 and even longer in some cases.

Myth #3: You can tell if you have it.

Myth: HPV always has symptoms.

Truth: It's often silent. That's why screening matters.

What You Can Do

1. Book Regular Cervical Screenings - In the UK, these are offered every 3-5 years up to age 64. Don't skip them, especially if you've had abnormal results before.

2. Ask About the HPV Vaccine = Still under 45 and unvaccinated? You may be eligible. Speak to your GP.

3. Support Your Immunity:

   a. Nutrition: Think berries, leafy greens, turmeric, citrus fruits.

   b. Movement: Gentle daily activity like walking or yoga.

   c. Sleep: Prioritise rest and recovery.

   d. Hydration: Flush toxins, support cellular health.

The Press-Pulsate-Pause Method™ for Cervical & Immune Health

(Refer to Chapter 3 for full instructions)

- **Spleen 6 三阴交 (Sān Yīn Jiāo)**
    - Place four fingers above your inner ankle bone, on the inside of your leg. You'll feel a tender spot just behind the shin bone - that's the one.
    - Supports your immune system, reproductive health, and hormone regulation.

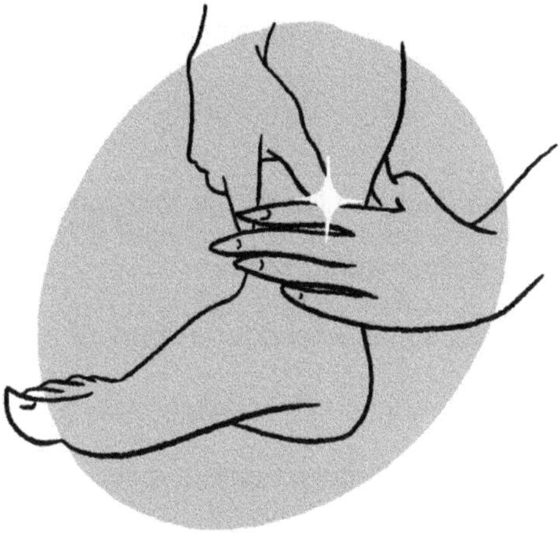

AcuWarrior™ Tip: Spleen 6 is a true multitasker and is often called the "meeting point of womanhood." It's one of the most powerful points for reproductive and immune health, but with great power comes a gentle warning: do not use this point during pregnancy, as it can stimulate uterine activity.

AromaAcu Therapy™ - Your Essential Oil Allies for Cervical Support

(Refer to Chapter 3 for how to use oils safely)

Recommended oils:

- Lavender - Calming, supportive of pelvic tension release and emotional ease.
- Tea Tree - Natural antimicrobial, supportive for vaginal and immune health (external use only).
- Frankincense - Cellular regeneration, grounding, encourages connection to the womb space.

Important Note (from one woman to another): Please do not apply essential oils inside the vagina or on tampons. No matter what TikTok tells you. Even natural oils can disrupt your delicate internal microbiome or cause serious irritation. Your cervix is sacred. Let's support it with respect, not risk.

Healing Breath Ritual for Grounding After Difficult News

Whether you've received unexpected results from your smear test, felt dismissed at your appointment, or are simply carrying too much - come home to yourself.

Ritual steps:

1. Sit upright with your feet flat on the floor, uncrossed and rooted. Place both hands gently over your lower abdomen, just below the navel, over your womb space.
2. Inhale softly through the nose for a count of 4.
3. Hold for 2.
4. Exhale slowly through the mouth for a count of 6
5. Repeat for 2 minutes, allowing your hands to feel warm and connected to your pelvic centre.

This breath pattern soothes your nervous system, reduces the body's stress response, and helps re-centre you after emotional overwhelm - especially when it relates to your cervical or reproductive health.

Your womb holds wisdom and this breath helps you hear it.

Don't skip smear tests, even if you're postmenopausal.

Boost your immune system with food, movement, and sleep.

Use AromaAcu Therapy™ to support stress relief.

If anxious, speak to your GP and a trusted practitioner - you're not alone.

Contact me for guidance - online or in-clinic support is available.

Final Myth-Busting Thought

Sometimes the most empowering thing you can do is ask better questions.

What belief are you ready to unlearn today?

Affirmation

"I am informed, empowered, and unapologetically taking control of my health."

Gratitude Prompt

Which myth did you once believe and what truth felt like a deep exhale as you let it go? Take a moment to honour the version of you who carried that misinformation. She was doing her best with what she knew. Now, thank yourself for choosing clarity over confusion, and truth over noise.

Knowledge is power. And you're reclaiming it.

Persian Wisdom

"The wound is the place where the light enters you."

زخم، جاییست که نور وارد می‌شود

Transliteration: Zakhm, jâyist keh noor vâred mishavad.

Meaning: What once felt like confusion or pain can become a portal to deeper understanding. Don't dismiss the myths you once believed. They brought you here, to this place of awakening.

Let's Keep Talking: *Heard a myth that made you roll your eyes or second-guess your body? Tag me using* **#PocketPeri** *and mention @AcuCareClinicUK - I'd love to hear the myths you've busted, the truths that landed, and the one thing you'll never believe again.*

Next Up: *A bonus chapter straight from my heart (and future book - wink wink). Your sneak peek into the next evolution of emotional skin therapy and embodied beauty.*

THE BONUS CHAPTER!

CHAPTER 19

Beauty & Wellness

The Art of Effortless Care

We've explored hormones, emotions, skin health, and all the surprising ways PeriMenopause shows up. Now? It's time for a little luxury. The kind that doesn't need filters, just intention.

You've earned this. Not because you pushed through, but because rest, ritual, and radiance are your birthright - not a reward.

This chapter isn't about anti-ageing. It's about anti-burnout. Effortless beauty, rooted in pleasure, presence, and a bit of Persian wisdom. It's time to glow on your terms.

Simple Self-Care Tips for Everyday Glow

Because beauty isn't about perfection, it's about presence. These daily rituals are designed to nourish your skin, recharge your energy, and remind you that self-care doesn't need to be complicated to be powerful.

Morning Refresh

Start the day with intention, not intensity.

- Spritz your face with pure rosewater. It's like a floral alarm clock for tired skin.
- Gently massage your moisturiser in upward strokes. This boosts circulation and tells your nervous system: We're safe. We're glowing. We've got this.
- Optional: Add a touch of Gua Sha if you've got a few extra minutes. (Want to learn the technique without harming your skin barrier? Join one of my workshops for a full demo or if you're after a quick version, head to Chapter 16: Feel Good to Look Good and scan the QR code in the relevant section.)

AcuWarrior™ Reminder: This isn't "anti-ageing", it's pro-glow.

Insider Tip: I craft a bespoke Persian Rose Mist Spray (100% pure rose water) tailored to each skin type. It's a clinic favourite, blending traditional care with modern skin wisdom. (Curious? Ask me about it during an online session or face-to-face visit.)

Midday Reset

When the afternoon slump hits, don't reach for another coffee. Reset instead.

- Inhale a drop of lavender or peppermint oil on a tissue or cotton wool. It helps release tension and perks up your senses.
- If your skin's flagging, press a cool chamomile tea-soaked cloth over your face for a quick refresh.

The Press-Pulsate-Pause Method™: (Refer to Chapter 3 for full instructions)

- **Large Intestine 4 合谷 (Hé Gŭ)**
    - In the web between thumb and index finger for a 60-second energy boost.
    - Avoid LI4 if you're pregnant or trying to conceive. It's a powerful, stimulating, point.

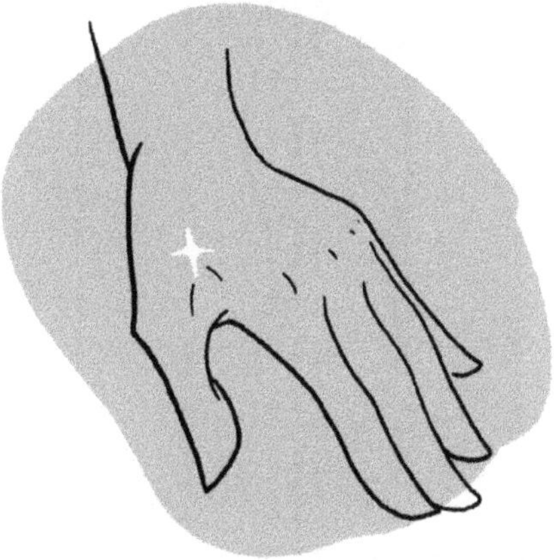

AcuWarrior™ Reminder: Self-care isn't selfish, it's smart biology.

Evening Wind-Down

Evenings are your time to shift gears from go-mode to glow-mode.

- After cleansing, mix 1 drop of lemon essential oil into 1 tablespoon of organic olive or coconut oil (a clean shot glass works well). Gently apply to your temples and/or soles of your feet for a refreshing, tension-releasing effect.

Safety Note: Lemon oil is highly photosensitive. Use only in the evening and ensure it's well diluted. If you're on any medication, check with a qualified professional before use.

The Press-Pulsate-Pause Method™: (Refer to Chapter 3 for full instructions)

- **Kidney 1 涌泉 (Yǒng Quán)**
    - On the sole of the foot, just below the ball, with a nourishing cream to calm your nervous system and promote deeper rest.

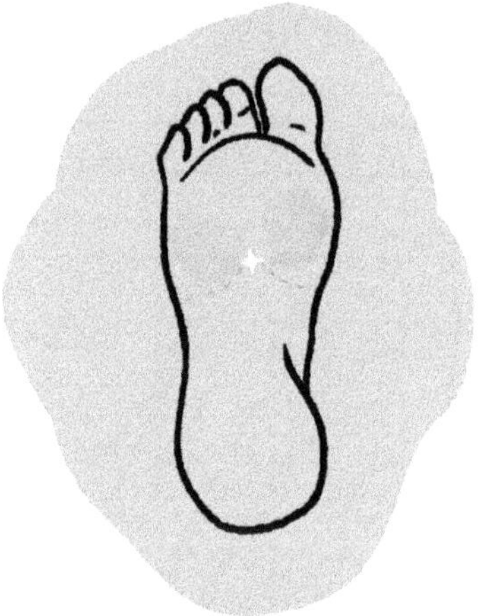

Ditch synthetic candles. Light a natural soy-based candle scented with pure essential oils like lavender, neroli, or rose. Your hormones will thank you.

AcuWarrior™ Reminder: Your skin doesn't need a filter, it needs a ritual.

AromaAcu Therapy™ - Beauty That Begins with Balance

Effortless beauty isn't just what you apply. It's how you feel.

AromaAcu Therapy™ blends the calming effects of aromatherapy with the energetic rebalancing of acupressure. It's not just for hormone balance or sleep, it's your secret weapon for glow, grace, and groundedness.

Time of Day	Essential Oil	Press-Pulsate-Pause Method™ Point	Why It Works
Morning	Peppermint or Lemon	Stomach 36	Boosts energy, supports circulation, and awakens tired skin
Midday	Rosemary or Eucalyptus	Large Intestine 4	Releases tension, improves clarity, and refreshes complexion
Evening	Lavender or Chamomile	Liver 3	Calms emotions, supports detox, and softens puffiness
Before Bed	Ylang Ylang or Rose	Kidney 1	Grounds the nervous system, promotes deep rest, and rejuvenates from within

(Refer to Chapter 3 for guidance)

*Avoid Large Intestine 4 if pregnant or trying to conceive.

AcuWarrior™ Tip: This ritual isn't vanity. It's vitality. Beauty isn't skin-deep when you treat your nervous system with the same attention you give your moisturiser.

DIY Beauty From Your Kitchen

Because your skin deserves ingredients you can actually pronounce.

You don't need a 12-step routine or luxury brands. Sometimes, the most comforting care starts with a teaspoon and a kitchen cupboard.

This won't beat a proper personalised blend, but it's such a nice little pause in a busy week and, honestly, mixing it up feels a bit like self-care alchemy. Think of it as active meditation with a splash of fun.

Overnight Glow Mask

A gentle kitchen remedy to revive dull or tired skin.

Ingredients:

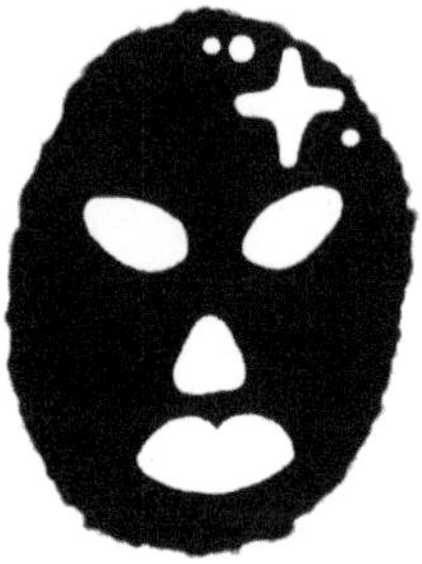

- 1 tsp organic honey (natural humectant to draw in moisture).
- 1 tsp Greek yoghurt (mild exfoliant + soothing probiotic).
- Optional: ½ tsp ground oats (for extra softness).

How to use:

Mix into a creamy paste. After cleansing, apply a light layer to your face (avoiding eyes). Leave on for 10-15 mins, rinse gently with warm water, and follow with your usual night cream or facial oil.

Safety Note: If you've got super-sensitive or reactive skin (eczema, rosacea, etc.), patch-test first or skip the oats. Natural doesn't always mean irritation-free, so listen to your skin.

AcuWarrior™ Tip: Think of this as your Sunday-night skin hug. A sweet, simple ritual and if your skin's asking for more? That's where custom blends come in.

Nourishing Lip Balm

Keep your lips soft, smooth, and kissably hydrated.

Ingredients:

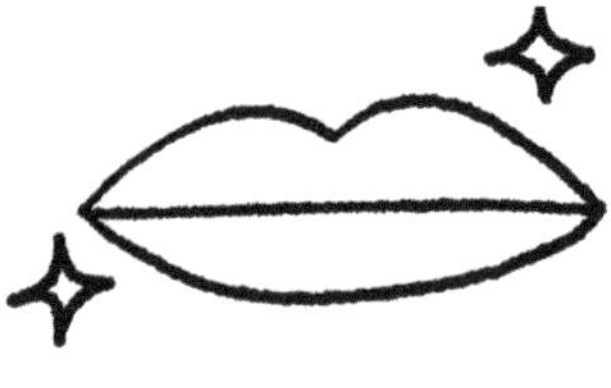

- 1 tbsp organic coconut oil.
- 1 drop pure vanilla extract.

How to make:

Pop the coconut oil into a small heatproof bowl and gently melt it (a quick 20-30 seconds over a bowl of hot water or a short microwave burst does the trick). Stir in the vanilla until it's fully blended.

How to use:

Pour into a little tin or pot and let it set at room temperature (or speed things up in the fridge if you're impatient). Swipe on whenever your lips feel dry or when you just fancy a tiny moment of self-care.

Bonus points if you hum your favourite tune while making it. DIY beauty is meant to be fun, not fussy.

Pro-Ageing: Celebrate Your Story

Let's make one thing clear: ageing isn't the enemy. Burnout is. Shame is. But age? Age is your evolution.

Mindset Reset: Ditch "anti-ageing". You're not here to erase time. You're here to own it. Every line, every laugh crease, every shift in your skin tells a story. Yours.

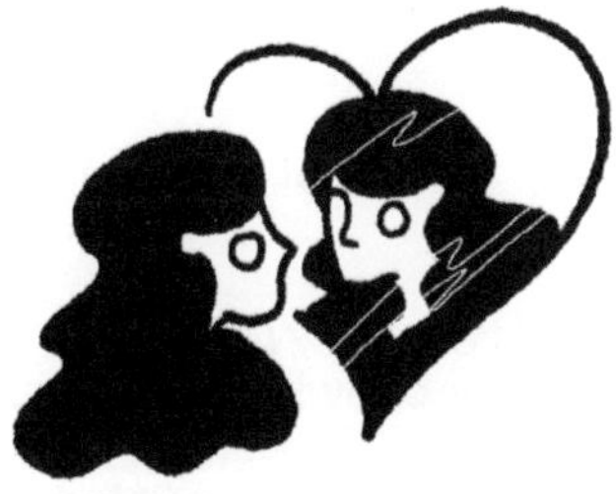

Skincare is now self-care: Think of each cleanse, each oil, each massage as a quiet love letter to yourself. You're not trying to turn back the clock, you're tuning into your body's rhythm.

AcuWarrior™ Tip: Confidence is the best foundation you'll ever wear. And it doesn't come in a bottle. It comes from finally caring more about how you feel, not how you're seen.

Healing Breath Ritual to Glow From the Inside Out

This ritual is as much for your nervous system as it is for your skin. Think of it as a mini facial for your soul.

Ritual steps:

1. Sit comfortably, shoulders relaxed, hands resting lightly on your cheeks or jawline.

2. Inhale slowly through your nose for 4 counts, imagining soft light filling your face and skin.

3. Hold for 2 counts, letting that glow "sink in."

4. Exhale gently through your mouth for 6 counts, releasing tension from your jaw, forehead, and mind.

5. Repeat for 2 minutes, keeping your touch gentle and loving.

AcuWarrior™ Tip: Pair this with your evening skincare. Breath + ritual = double the radiance.

Affirmation

"My beauty reflects the care I give myself - simple, intentional, and full of love."

Gratitude Prompt

"What's one small thing I did today that felt like true self-care, not a chore, but a gift to myself?"

Write it down. Big or tiny, it all counts. Notice how it made you feel, and let that gratitude settle into your body like a quiet glow.

AcuWarrior™ Reminder: True radiance isn't bottled. It's breathed, felt, lived. The creams and oils? Just the cherry on top.

Persian Wisdom

"Patience polishes the soul."

صبوری روح را جلا می‌دهد

Transliteration: Sābouri rooh rā jalā mīdehad

Meaning: True beauty doesn't come from rushing. It's the glow of a woman who's allowed herself space, grace, and time to unfold. Like polishing a gem, self-care takes consistency, not perfection.

Final Thought

The most powerful kind of beauty doesn't demand effort. It invites presence. You don't need a new routine - just a renewed relationship with yourself.

So here's to the real radiance. The kind that doesn't age, doesn't apologise, and doesn't play by the rules.

Keep it simple. Keep it soulful.

And remember: filters fade but rituals? They leave a glow that lasts.

AcuWarrior™ Nudge: "Your glow isn't hiding in a jar, it's hiding in your pause. Two minutes of breath, touch, or presence a day keeps the burnout away."

Let's Keep Talking: *Your glow isn't just skin-deep, it's story-deep.Tag me using* **#PocketPeri** *and mention @AcuCareClinicUK with your Sunday-night skin hug, your two-minute ritual, or that tiny act of self-kindness that made you feel radiant.*

Next Up: *Whether you're a partner, daughter, son, or colleague this next chapter is for you. It's a practical, heartfelt guide on how to show up for the women in your life as they navigate PeriMenopause.*

CHAPTER 20

Supporting Women

A Guide for Loved Ones

This is the chapter to share. Read it out loud.
Leave it open on the kitchen table.
Screenshot it for your group chat.

Why This Chapter Matters

This chapter is for you, the partner, daughter, son, friend, or colleague who cares about someone navigating PeriMenopause. Maybe you stumbled upon this book, or maybe she passed it to you with a hopeful smile and the words: "This might help you understand." Either way, thank you for being here.

PeriMenopause isn't always easy to explain. It can be confusing, overwhelming, and - let's be honest - awkward to talk about, but this chapter is your invitation to lean in with curiosity, not fear. It's your roadmap for connection, even when the road gets bumpy.

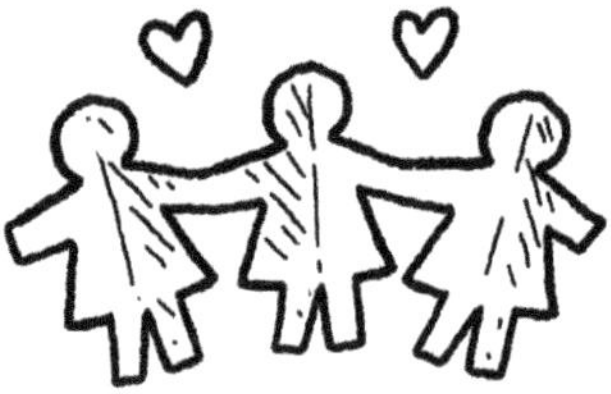

When It Clicked

"When My Husband Finally Got It"

Sarah had been feeling emotionally isolated. Her partner kept telling her to "calm down" or "go for a run." One night, after yet another miscommunication, she left a few pages of this book open on the kitchen table. The next morning, he came over, hugged her, and said: "I didn't realise what this really was. I'm sorry I haven't been more present."

Now, they check in weekly. Not perfectly but honestly. That changed everything.

What's an Affirmation and Why Are We Starting Here?

An affirmation is a powerful, present-tense statement that reminds us of what's possible. We begin this chapter with one because it sets the tone, not just for the reader, but for everyone involved. It helps ground us in empathy, presence, and intention. So before we dive in, take a deep breath. Whether you're the one going through it or the one supporting her, let this affirmation be your shared anchor.

Affirmation

"We may not always understand each other, but we choose patience, love, and presence. Together, we're stronger."

Understanding PeriMenopause

PeriMenopause isn't just about hot flushes, that "time of the month", and mood swings. It's about identity, energy, memory, confidence, and sometimes, loss.

It can look like:

- Fatigue so deep it feels like walking through mud.
- Forgetting names mid-sentence and wondering if you're losing your mind.
- Feeling anxious or flat for no clear reason.
- Wanting space but not rejection.
- Craving closeness but feeling too tired for it.

It's physical. It's emotional. It's hormonal. And most importantly, it's real.

Many women going through it feel invisible. Or misunderstood. Or labelled as "too sensitive." That's why this chapter exists to build bridges of empathy.

How to Be a Supportive Partner, Friend, or Family Member

For Partners:

- Listen without trying to fix. She doesn't need solutions, she needs to feel heard.
- Support her without needing credit. If the bins are overflowing, take them out. If she's quiet, sit beside her. Your presence speaks volumes.
- Redefine intimacy. Touch doesn't have to lead to sex. A hand on her back, a long hug, or just holding hands can be deeply healing.

For Friends:

- Be her safe space. Let her vent without needing to solve anything. A cheeky drink or a walk-and-talk might be all she needs.

- Check in regularly. Even a quick “Thinking of you today” message can go a long way.

For Family Members:

- Don’t dismiss her experience. Avoid phrases like, “It’s just your hormones,” or “You’re too young for menopause.”

- Be patient with her energy. She might not attend every gathering or reply to every message and that doesn’t mean she doesn’t care.

For Colleagues and Work Friends:

PeriMenopause doesn’t clock out at 9 a.m. Brain fog, temperature swings, or emotional shifts may show up in meetings or at the desk next to you. What helps?

- Compassion over criticism.

- Flexibility over judgement.

- She’s not making excuses - she’s managing a hormonal recalibration.

For Children and Teens:

She’s still your mum, auntie, or big sister, just maybe a little more tired or emotional sometimes. It’s not your fault, and it’s not about you. A hug, a hand, a “How can I help?” can make her day.

What NOT to Say

Sometimes we mean well but our words miss the mark. Here are a few phrases to rethink:

“You were fine yesterday!” - PeriMenopause symptoms can shift by the hour. Trust what she’s feeling today.

“You just need to go for a walk.” - Exercise helps - but so does compassion.

“You’re being hormonal.” - Translation: “Your feelings don’t count.” Let’s not go there.

Try This Instead: Compassionate Communication Tools

Active Listening. Nod. Make eye contact. Reflect back what she says. "So you're feeling overwhelmed about work and your body. I hear you."

Ask, don't assume. "What do you need today?" is always better than guessing.

Use "I" Statements. "I feel concerned when I see you struggling. How can I help?"

AcuWarrior™ Tip: When in doubt, don't fix. Just sit, listen, and offer a warm drink. Sometimes the best response is: "That sounds tough. I'm here." Silence can be sacred. So can snacks.

Create a PeriSupport Kit

Whether you live together or check in from afar, here are a few thoughtful things to keep on hand:

- Weighted blanket - Calms the nervous system.
- Notebook or journal - A space for her thoughts (or yours!).
- Feel-good playlist - Co-create a soundtrack that lifts the mood.
- Join our community playlist: PocketPeri - The Empowerment Mix on Spotify. It's a co-created space for music that lifts, soothes, and empowers you through every phase. Submit your favourite tracks via @AcuCareClinicUK on Instagram.

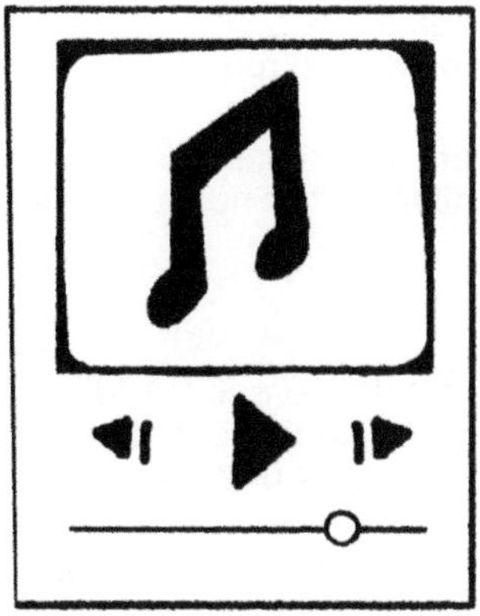

- Comfort food - We're not anti-sugar, we're pro-survival.
- Essential oils - Try inhaling lavender or peppermint using the damp cotton wool method.
- Box breathing - Inhale for 4, hold for 4, exhale for 4, hold for 4. Repeat for 2 minutes together.

You don't need all of these. One or two thoughtful items go a long way.

Healing Breath Ritual for Togetherness

When words feel too much or not enough, let breath do the talking. This simple ritual helps you reconnect without needing to fix or explain.

1. Sit comfortably. Hold hands if it feels natural.
2. Close your eyes and breathe in slowly for 4 seconds. Feel your body soften.
3. Hold the breath for 4. Let the pause be peaceful.
4. Exhale gently for 4. Release the day.
5. Hold again for 4. Let stillness settle.
6. Repeat for 4 rounds. It's not about perfection. It's about presence.

Solo option: If you're reading this alone, place one hand over your heart and the other over your belly. You're holding yourself and that counts too.

AcuWarrior™ Reminder: "Connection doesn't always come from words. Sometimes, it's shared silence that heals the most."

Gratitude Prompt

Take a quiet moment and ask yourself the following: what did I learn about her (or myself) by reading this chapter? What's one small way I can show more patience, love, or understanding this week?

Gratitude isn't just for the person going through PeriMenopause. It's for you too. Acknowledge the care you're giving and the connection you're building - these small acts create lasting bridges.

(If you're reading this aloud, pause for a breath together. Let the gratitude land between you.)

Persian Wisdom

مهربانی پلی‌ست که دل‌ها را به هم پیوند می‌دهد

"Kindness is the bridge that connects hearts." - Persian Proverb

Transliteration: Mehrabāni pol-i-st keh del-hā rā beh ham peyvand midahad

Meaning: True support isn't about grand gestures - it's the small, loving actions repeated daily. A warm tone. A shared silence. A kind word at the right moment. That's what builds unshakeable bonds.

Final Thought

You don't have to understand it all to show up with love. You just have to keep showing up. To the readers who handed this chapter to someone they love - bravo. To the loved ones who are reading it - thank you. This is how change happens. One conversation, one act of care, one shared page at a time.

***Let's Keep Talking**: Conversations like this don't end on one page. Tag me using **#PocketPeri** and mention @AcuCareClinicUK. I'd love to hear how this chapter opened up a conversation in your home, your relationship, or even within yourself.*

***Next Up**: You've made it through the science, the symptoms, the sass, and the soul work. But we're not quite done.*

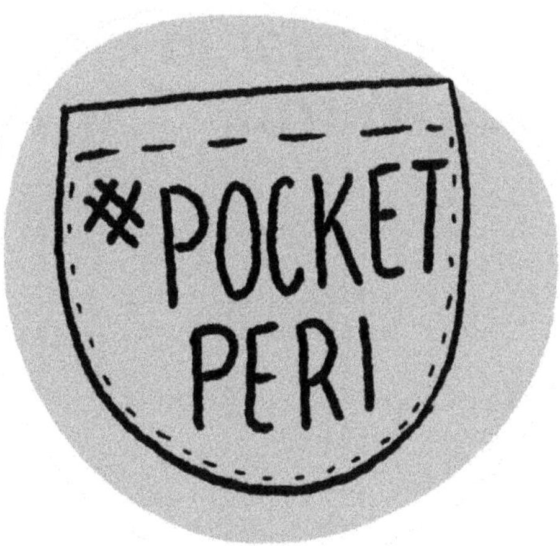

CHAPTER 21

Final Words

A Letter to the
AcuWarrior™ *in You*

Dear AcuWarrior™,

You've made it.

Not just to the end of this book but through the countless days when your body surprised you, your mind challenged you, and your heart cracked open in unexpected ways.

Back in Chapter 1, we planted a seed. A quiet knowing that your story matters. That you're not "just hormonal" or "going through a phase", you're evolving. Page by page, symptom by symptom, chapter by chapter, you've been reclaiming your power.

This final chapter isn't here to wrap things up with a neat bow. It's here to honour everything messy, beautiful, misunderstood, and miraculous about your PeriMenopause journey.

Because this chapter belongs to you.

A Letter for the You Who's Still Figuring It Out

There will be days when you feel strong. There will be days when you feel everything but, and both are okay. You are not defined by how productive, cheerful, or composed you appear.

You are defined by your decision to show up - again and again - for yourself.

You're the woman who kept reading. Who paused when the tears came. Who laughed when a symptom sounded all too familiar.

You're the woman who whispered "yes" under her breath when a truth finally landed.

You're the woman who now knows that she's not alone.

That is power. Not performative power but the quiet kind that lives in your pulse. In your rituals. In your voice.

You are an AcuWarrior™. Not because you fought, but because you softened. You dared to care for yourself in a world that taught you to ignore the signs.

Choosing the Right Support: Acupuncture & Beyond

If this book has sparked curiosity about Traditional Chinese Medicine (TCM) and Acupuncture, you're not alone. This is a complete system of medicine. It's clinically grounded, globally respected, and has been used for centuries to support women's health. If you feel drawn to explore it, I encourage you to find a practitioner who is not only qualified but someone who makes you feel heard, safe, and supported.

Here's what I recommend to look for:

- A degree-trained Acupuncture Practitioner (i.e. Acupuncturist) registered with a reputable body (e.g. the British Acupuncture Council in the UK or who are recommended by the NHS).
- Someone who listens - really listens - before offering treatment.
- A setting where you feel safe, respected, and empowered.

I offer complimentary 20-minute consultations (online or in person) to help women find the right path, even if that path isn't with me. Because it's not about me. It's about you.

Your Journey Continues With or Without This Book in Your Hands

Whether you dog-eared pages, highlighted rituals, or simply read in quiet reflection, know this:

You've begun a lifelong dialogue with your body. Let that conversation stay open. You don't need to rush to the next chapter in life.

But when you're ready:

- I run seasonal self-care retreats and workshops.
- I create PeriMenopause support kits designed with ritual and relief in mind.
- I offer holistic sessions that bring together acupuncture, acupressure, and AromaAcu Therapy™.

You can explore more at: www.acucareclinic.co.uk/next

And when you're in the mood for soul-soothing music? Join our community playlist: **#PocketPeri** - The Empowerment Mix on Spotify. It's a co-created space, just submit your favourite tracks via @AcuCareClinicUK on Instagram.

Because healing isn't just about science. It's also about songs, stories, and shared spaces.

Gratitude Prompt

Take a deep breath, pause, and place your left hand over your heart. Ask what's one thing this journey has taught you about yourself that you didn't know before? Who or what are you grateful for in helping you reach this moment - no matter how small?

Let that gratitude ripple through your breath. This isn't the end of a book. It's the beginning of a new relationship with yourself.

Persian Wisdom

"She sat with her pain, until it turned into power."

نشست با دردش، تا به قدرت تبدیل شد

Transliteration: Neshast bâ dardesh, tâ be ghodrat tabdil shod.

Meaning: True strength doesn't always roar. Sometimes, it's found in the quiet act of staying with yourself long enough to transform.

A Final Affirmation

Before you close this chapter, pause and breathe these words into your body:

"I am not broken. I am becoming. Today, I honour every step I've taken to understand myself. I thank those who stood beside me and I extend love to the woman I've become."

Say it aloud. Whisper it. Write it on a sticky note. This isn't just an affirmation, it's a reminder. You've earned this moment, and there are so many more waiting for you.

And one final whisper before you go: You were never "losing yourself." You were returning home. To you. To your rhythm. To your radiance.

With love, always,

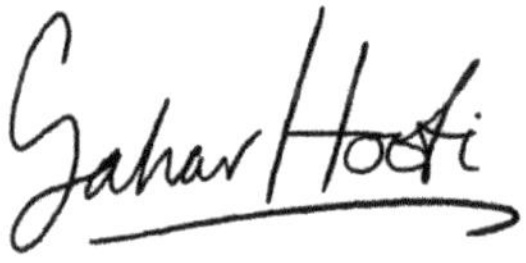

Your fellow AcuWarrior™ and guide on this wild, wonderful, ride through PeriMenopause.

@ACUCARE_CLINIC_UK

ACKNOWLEDGEMENTS

Books don't write themselves - despite what Google might suggest! This one came to life through the love, patience, wisdom, and encouragement of so many people. To name you all here is both a joy and a responsibility, and I hope these words reflect even a fraction of the gratitude I carry.

To my sister Roxana Hooti, my designer and publisher, founder of Brut Magazine, and an author in her own right. Keeping this book a passion project within the family is one of my proudest choices. To Leanne Curran - editor, patient, book coach, and my on-call calm voice during panic moments - and to her mum, Julie, who cheered me on from the very start. To my amazing friend Catherine Burt, for generous PR and book launch ideas, proofreading, guidance, and encouragement. To Charley at Teams Local, for the videos, QR codes, and tech support. To Lulu, who connected dots (thanks to Birute's introduction) and helped me keep going. And to Sara Annovi, photographer from Fuerteventura who captured me at the place where I finished my very first draft.

To Birute Thomas, owner of Studio B Collective, connector of people, and an inspiration in her own right. Thank you for believing in me, for opening doors, and for reminding me what true community looks like.

To Helena Sterne, for mentorship and friendship; to Shaa Wasmund, who pushed me to think bigger; to Chris Richards and Pete Scott, for your past mentorship; and to Stephanie Chivers & Matt Thomas for your coaching along the way. To my boxing coaches, Gemma and Zainab, for keeping me sane. To Linda, my saxophone teacher, for cheering me on (even when the sax had to take a back seat). And to Sarah Chamberlain (Chaulk Education), Mollie Hogan (Mollie Hair), and Olga Herrmann (Fuerteventura), for hair support along the way.

To Wilson Lu, Elena Diana, Catherine Burt, Aina Šutka, Claire Bolsover (for giving me the honour of being "Auntie" to your beautiful children), Suzy, Zoe Raluca, Sam, Susan & Ali Mahinfar, Pat & Simon, Sophia Husbands, Claire, Max, Mark & Emma, Daoud V, Barbara Light, Heather, Elizabeth, Roxane and Sinead. Thank you all for being my cheerleaders in your own ways. What I love about our friendships is that we've always got each other's backs, no matter what.

To my mum - who came through her transition like a queen and inspired me to write this book. To my dad - who, through his hobby of writing songs and stories, encouraged me to write as well. To my siblings - Sophia, Sam, Susan, and Roxana - for sharing the long journey of education and resilience, and to my brothers-in-law Kevin and Ashley, for being part of that support system too. To my nephew Noah - for bringing such zest to life and reminding me not to sweat the small stuff. To my cousins and extended family - for their support from afar, even though continents separate us. To my Iranian friends - both those still in Iran and those now scattered around the world - thank you for your love, encouragement, and solidarity across distance. To my Gareth - my anchor and voice of reason on the days I wanted to quit. You were there from day one , the moment I decided to actually write this book. And to my wider family, scattered across the world - living examples of courage and resilience.

To Zari, Hamid, Mona, Diana, Jane, and Jill - family friends who have always been there.

To Emily Barclay, who co-authored with me before this solo book, planted the seed for me to write my own, and gave me confidence when she invited me onto the Ideal Home Show panel in 2024 - a stepping stone to going solo in 2025. To the beautiful network of authors I've met along the way - it's been a joy to share this path with people walking a similar road, learning, encouraging, and cheering each other on. To Neil at Portsmouth City Council, for clarity and guidance as I rebuilt my clinic space after lockdown. To my local community - Southsea, Portsmouth, Waterlooville, Studio B Collective (Birute and all the kind colleagues here), and the Farmhouse Sanctuary (all kind colleagues, especially Naomi and Trevor) - for being my roots and wings. To Rosanna and Chris, for the sober rave events (Loud & Clear) that kept me sane and gave me something to look forward to. To Ellie Storey, my social media manager, for her support behind the scenes. To all my colleagues in the wellbeing space, and to those who supported me with nails, massages, acupuncture, skincare, and the little acts of kindness that carried me through. To everyone I consulted with - whether we worked together or not - your time and insight were invaluable.

To my patients - who tolerated my distracted "PeriBrain" moments and still encouraged me; many of you have become dear friends. To my social media community - your daily messages reminded me why this book matters. And to the BAcC Facebook support group, with my fellow admins Sandra and Colette, for your patience, encouragement, and solidarity.

To my teachers - every single one of you who shaped the way I think, the way I see the world, and the way I practise. To my patients once again - who have taught me just as much as I've ever taught them. And to the spirits of my loved ones - I felt your presence protecting me and guiding me throughout this journey.

There were moments I almost gave up - especially during difficult world events that weighed heavily. Thank you to everyone who held me in those moments - with compassion, cups of tea, and quiet presence. Your care helped me keep going.

Above all, I thank God. Through this process, I became more aware of who I am - my soul, my awareness, my spirit. That awareness deepened my compassion not only for my patients, but for my family, my friends, for strangers, and, perhaps most importantly, for myself. It isn't a boast, just a quiet lesson in kindness. Life is short, and whether or not you believe in an afterlife, why not make our time on this earth more pleasurable, more mindful, and more filled with self-love? That is what I hope this book inspires.

"دوش ایرد یهگناو ،ددرگ عمج هرطقهرطق"

Transliteration: Qatreh qatreh jam gardad, vangahi daryā shavad

Meaning: "Drop by drop, it gathers - and then it becomes the sea." Small, steady steps create vast legacies. This book is the ocean born of countless drops of love, patience, and encouragement.

And lastly - I thank myself. For not giving up when it would have been easier to quit. For carrying this through, drop by drop. If this has started to sound like an Oscar speech, well… at least there are no tears or awkward music cues to cut me off. Just gratitude - pure, stubborn, Peri-powered gratitude. And if I have forgotten your name, please forgive me. Blame it on PeriBrain, not my heart.

BOOK LAUNCH LOVE

At the time of finalising this book, the launch event hadn't yet happened - but the planning certainly had! I forgot just how much work goes into organising a celebration like this. What I didn't forget was the kindness, community, and behind-the-scenes brilliance that held it all together.

To Danni at Panero Lounge, Southsea, thank you for offering the perfect venue (and for your patience through my many questions!).

To Lulu, director of Love Southsea, my fabulous host, for bringing sparkle, style, and Southsea soul.

To Lauren (hair), Ruby (nails), and everyone who helped me feel my best on the day - it's the little touches that made a big difference. A special thank you to Freya Rose London for the beautiful jewellery I wore on the night - pieces that made the occasion feel even more special.

To the incredible coaches and mentors who guided me throughout this process - and to Roxana Hooti and Cat Charlton (and her amazing team) for walking beside me with clarity, heart, and fierce vision.

To Catherine Burt, again, for your generous PR ideas, helping with event planning, prep, hosting, and constant encouragement.

To Jo and Caroline, the brilliant PR team working with the British Acupuncture Council, thank you for inviting me to be featured for Acupuncture Awareness Wee - an honour I cherish, especially as this book launches hot on the heels of World PeriMenopause Day (11th October) and World Menopause Day (18th October).

Launching this book on the 20th of October 2025 felt like the natural next step - a way to keep the conversation going, carry the momentum forward, and remind women everywhere that this phase of life deserves a voice, a spotlight, and a community.

To everyone who offered help, shared words of encouragement, moved mountains behind the scenes, or simply held space for me - thank you. The love, generosity, and support around this launch have been overwhelmingly beautiful. Whether you could be there in person or cheered me on from afar, your energy is forever woven into this moment.

And it goes without saying - my deepest gratitude, overflowing with love, to my family, my closest friends, my partner, and of course my wonderful patients.

APPENDIX

- *GenM Invisibility Report; Menopause Support UK; Grand View Research 2024) https://www.grandviewresearch.com/industry-analysis/menopause-market

- **https://www.berkshirehealthcare.nhs.uk/media/109514306/2-adhd-guide-adhd-in-women.pdf - Berkshire Healthcare NHS Trust

- ***Registered member of the British Acupuncture Council

- Visit AcuCare Clinic for more information, and to explore Sahar's products and retreats. https://www.acucareclinic.co.uk

Recommended Oils:

- Cinnamon
- Clary Sage
- Eucalyptus
- Fennel
- Frankincense
- Geranium
- Ginger
- Jasmine
- Lavender
- Lemon
- Orange
- Peppermint
- Petitgrain
- Roman Chamomile
- Rose
- Rosemary
- Sweet Orange
- Tea Tree

ABOUT THE AUTHOR

I'm Sahar Hooti, BSc (Hons), ***MBAcC - a Traditional & Western degree-trained Acupuncture Practitioner, Aromatherapist, Women's Hormonal Health & Skin Specialist and a qualified educator with an Ofqual-regulated teaching certification. Born in Iran during the Iran-Iraq War in 1981 and raised between Iran, Australia, and England, I've spent over 20 years working in holistic health, skin care, and Traditional Chinese Medicine.

I founded AcuCare Clinic UK to give women practical, science-backed tools to navigate PeriMenopause naturally. Out of that work (and my own journey through PeriMenopause) came the Press-Pulsate-Pause Method™ - my signature Advanced Acupressure technique - and AromaAcu Therapy™, blending aromatherapy with acupressure to support body and mind.

My Persian roots are woven through everything I do. The women who raised me - my mother, grandmother, and aunts - taught me that healing is as much about story and soul as it is about science. You'll find their wisdom in these pages, alongside modern clinical insight.

Alongside my clinic, I've been featured in the press for my pioneering work in women's health and skincare, spoken at national events such as the Ideal Home Show, and shared my expertise through workshops, retreats, and community education.

Outside the clinic and away from my writing desk, you'll usually find me boxing to shake off stress, blasting out tunes on my saxophone (loudly and badly most days - but it brings me pure joy!), dancing my heart out to DnB, and, most importantly, soaking up quality time with my loved ones - especially my little cutie of a nephew, Noah.

This book is my love letter to every woman navigating PeriMenopause. It's not just a guide - it's a reminder that you are not broken. You are becoming.

For media and events: AcuCareClinic.co.uk

www.ingramcontent.com/pod-product-compliance
Ingram Content Group UK Ltd.
Pitfield, Milton Keynes, MK11 3LW, UK
UKHW041915091025
463792UK00005B/18

9 781919 267005